Acceptance and Commitment Therapy for Chronic Pain

Dedication

To my favorite young women, Emma, my daughter, and Jenny, my niece, along with all of my female students. May this book serve as a source of inspiration for you as young women to have the courage to take a step forward in the light of your own unique vitality, show your greatness and by doing so make your special contribution towards bettering our world. (JD)

To my mom and dad, Barbara and Jim,
for their unending support and love (KGW)

To the students, who were willing to accept their own pain in order to help patients live a valued life with theirs (CL)

To Jacque, Happiness is Love (SCH)

Acceptance and Commitment Therapy for Chronic Pain

JoAnne Dahl
Uppsala University
Kelly G. Wilson
University of Mississippi
Carmen Luciano
University of Almería
Steven C. Hayes
University of Nevada, Reno

CONTEXT PRESS

Reno, NV

Publisher's Note

This publication is designed to provide accurate and authoritative information in regard to the subject matter covered. It is sold with the understanding that the publisher is not engaged in rendering psychological, financial, legal, or other professional services. If expert assistance or counseling is needed, the services of a competent professional should be sought.

Distributed in Canada by Raincoast Books

Copyright © 2005 Context Press
Context Press is a division of New Harbinger Publications, Inc.
5674 Shattuck Avenue
Oakland, CA 94609
www.newharbinger.com

All drawings and cover by Jonathan Dahl

Library of Congress Cataloging-in-Publication Data

Acceptance and commitment therapy for chronic pain / JoAnne Dahl ... [et al.].
p. cm.
   Includes bibliographical references.
   ISBN-13: 978-1-878978-52-3 (pbk.)
   ISBN-10: 1-878978-52-7 (pbk.)
 1. Chronic pain—Treatment. 2. Behavior therapy. I. Dahl, JoAnne, 1951-
   RB127.A24 2005
   616'.0472—dc22

                                        2005008039

Preface

The handbook you now have in your hands represents, for me, over 25 years of practical clinical and clinical research in rehabilitation medical centers trying to help clients who are "stuck" in chronic pain get "loose" and go on with their lives. The application of behavioral analysis on physical symptoms was a revolutionary development called behavior medicine that got started in the 1970's. It was radical because it actually entailed a paradigm shift from a mechanical medical model to a whole new conceptualization of illness which included the learning model. The principles of conditioning were now being combined with medical know-how into a synthesis model of treatment that really made a difference in helping people with chronic illness regain function and life quality. The greatest difference produced by this marriage of behavior therapy and medicine was the concept of *context*. According to the medical model, physical illness occurred within the body and was caused by some pathological process. Consequently, the aim of treatment was to find that pathology and alleviate it. What behavior analysis brought to the marriage was the concept that no symptom takes place in a vacuum. All physical symptoms are amenable to the principles of learning.

The radical difference shown in this new paradigm was that the probability of developing a chronic disability was not determined by the actual symptoms themselves but rather the conditioning or context. Subsequently behavior therapists within the medical units would "diagnose" using functional analyses of the context of the symptom. This was done together with the whole rehab team. The two-step analysis was used to hypothesize the context of what the classical conditioning took place from the start and how the operant conditioning developed mostly in the form of fear-avoidance of the symptoms. Subsequently, treatment aimed at "de-conditioning" the symptoms by means of exposure on all fronts. This implied that each rehab team member would work within this functional analysis context and aim at de-conditioning by means of exposure. The context of this de-conditioning process was usually fairly pre-set. Insurance companies or employers paying for the rehabilitation wanted the client back to work. The rehab team members, often educated within the medical model, had pretty firm ideas as how to get the client back on his or her feet and back to work. Physical therapists aimed at helping clients strengthen and relax muscles, gain a better physical fitness and regain normal movement patterns. Occupational therapists aimed at helping clients work more ergonomically and expose themselves to work-like activities. Social workers aimed at helping the client get started in getting back to work. The CBT psychologist led the team in exposure and often worked in groups helping the clients to increase social skills and use different cognitive techniques for reducing negative thoughts. This type of CBT multi-disciplinary program for chronic pain truly represents a giant step in how we conceptualize and treat chronic illness. Today, such programs are seen as the treatment of choice for chronic pain.

The application of Acceptance and Commitment Therapy for chronic illness generally and specially for chronic pain is, to my mind, the next giant development. Again, it has to do with the development of the concept of *context*. About five years ago, I attended a workshop by Kelly Wilson here in Sweden on ACT. Kelly was putting his finger on something in the ACT model that struck me as sorely missing from the CBT model of chronic pain as I had worked with it and seen it, in many places. Kelly spoke about the concept of using the client's values as the context of exposure and using the functional analysis even for the conceptualization and subsequent treatment of the client's language. Kelly also demonstrated a very different therapeutic posture than the sort of teacher/student positioning that I was used to within CBT.

If you look at the empirical studies evaluating the CBT multi-disciplinary treatment of chronic pain, there is relatively good evidence as to its effectiveness with respect especially to helping clients back to work. Why then, should we go on to something else, if this is working so well? A good hard look at what goes on in these clinics will help you to see why the ACT model "hit home" on a number of issues. First of all, several major scientific reviews have shown that the CBT model is more helpful than traditional medical treatments alone in helping getting clients back to work, but due to the multiple components of treatment, none have been able to shed light as to what is working. Also there are very few randomized controlled trials with adequate control conditions. A particularly difficult problem, with almost all of the evaluation studies done on CBT multi-disciplinary programs, is that the rehab physicians on these same units are in charge of the most important dependent variable, the disability certificate. There is a contract from the start from the insurance agencies sponsoring the rehabilitation that at the end of the treatment period, the sick certificate will be terminated. The end result is in fact defined from the start and what happens during that period may not be of much consequence. This is a sure way to get results! This somewhat "hidden" agenda is the source of much conflict between the rehab staff and the clients.

Try and picture this scene. The client with chronic pain comes to the rehab clinic because pain and resulting disability has stopped him or her from working and functionally generally. Consider also the fact that most persons with pain in the neck, back or shoulders never seek help at all and of those who do, most recover quickly or find that they have a progressive illness that needs attention. Those persons, who do not have a progressive illness, do not get better from the usual treatment and who get "stuck" in chronic pain and disability are those who come to rehab. Most often these individuals have already been treated with suspicion questioning the authenticity of the disability due to the fact that they have not improved as expected. They will also be aware of the social frowning on those who are seen as "cheating" the health insurance systems by simulating pain symptoms for the economic gains of disability payments. In our culture, any kind of pain that is not physical and associated with some organic pathology is under suspicion of not being "real". So, picture this individual, overwhelmed with pain symptoms, whose credibility is questioned by the health care system, employer, friends, and family, now being coerced into complying with a rehabilitation program.

The rehab team, on the other hand has about an 8-week period to fulfill their contract and get the person back to work. By means of the functional analysis the team creates a hypothesis regarding what types of activities, movements or situations that have been conditioned to pain. The treatment plan aims at de-conditioning these associations by means of exposure. The major problem facing the rehab staff is that the client is not on this wavelength and just the thought of exposure is aversive for this individual. Besides the fact that we are asking them to do things they are convinced will increase their already unbearable pain, we are also in a sense saying that they are wrong in their thinking. We are in essence saying that their pain is not "real", it is psychological. As if that weren't enough to set the stage for a poor therapeutic alliance, the insurance companies are standing behind the staff so that any non-compliance can result in loss of disability payment. You can imagine what types of behavior patterns these contingencies form. At worse, there is an atmosphere of "we" and "them" between the staff and the clients fighting for diametrically different goals. There is often conflict between the players, resulting in "burn out" among the staff and "pliance" or rule-governed compliance among the client. Clients do what they need to do half heartedly in order to please the insurance companies and never really integrate the rehabilitation efforts. Clients spend a lot of energy demonstrating pain and suffering and the rehab staff spends energy convincing and coaching the clients to expose them to pain. These programs are highly expensive due to all of the professionals in the team and number of inpatient hours for the client. Unless some progressive disease is discovered during the rehab time, the result of the rehabilitation time is the same regardless of how things go; disability payment is terminated and client goes back to work or on unemployment, permanent disability or social welfare.

As I listened to Kelly Wilson and read the first ACT book, I reflected over how the CBT model for rehabilitation of chronic pain could be developed in such as way so as to use the same principles of functional analysis and exposure that did not create aversion and resistance from the client and for the staff. How could we stand on the shoulders of those behavior therapists and cognitive behavior therapists who had paved the way into behavior medicine, carry forward these principles and do it in a way that was experienced as less aversive for all and create long-standing meaningful behavior changes?

The answer again was the conceptualization of *context*. In ACT as well as in all of the "third wave" behavior therapies the concept of context is developed from the more simplistic chains of fear-avoidance behavior to context on a higher human level. In this sense the functional analysis would not simply describe the immediate triggers and functions of chains of pain behavior but would examine the function of pain and fears of pain in a much wider context for each individual.

During the past five years I have radically changed rehabilitation programs along these lines in clinical settings and in a number of research projects. The programs described in this book show the same learning theory platform using the functional analysis as the basic guideline and exposure as the core treatment component. The difference is the how and the why. Using the clients' own values as the context to motivate behavior change is a brilliant idea. The goals of the treatment are no longer those of the insurance company and the staff members but belong within the context of the client. The job of the staff is to treat the client as an individual who is perfectly capable of choosing his or her own life and taking responsibility for it. The pressure is off the staff to coach, coerce or convince the client to expose themselves to aversive pain stimuli. The pressure is off the client to resist, be right, show pain symptoms, or maintain their position. The therapeutic relationship is now an alliance where both the staff and the client are working in the same direction. The client takes the lead and the rehab staff follows providing support only when asked for.

The other main difference in this ACT model for chronic pain is the functional analysis and treatment of client's language. Rather than working with dysfunctional thoughts associated with pain, which was done previously, ACT introduces a radically different approach far more consistent with functional analysis. Function rather than content of language including thoughts characterized all therapeutic interactions, which literally ended most all conflicts. Through a more general functional approach to all language and more specifically through what is called defusion exercises the staff and the client learn to observe thoughts as thoughts and examine their function rather than content. The message is that thoughts, feelings and pain sensations are phenomena beyond our control as is our reaction to them but we do have control over how we relate to and act towards them. In essence, this means that thoughts like "I can never go back to work with this pain" can be present at the same time as one takes steps to go back to work. The concept of acceptance here means that clients learn to accept phenomena which they have anyway and cannot control like pain sensations, thoughts, worries, fears about pain and put their energy in phenomena which they can control like their behavior. The aim of the ACT model in pain is creating flexibility around the client's stuckness in pain and building behavior repertoire towards valued life directions.

The conceptualization of chronic pain in the light of ACT and subsequent treatment models guidelines are presented in this book. Right from the start and all through the book you will follow Elisabeth in her struggle and recovery from chronic pain. Her story and her context contain most of the central core issues present for most clients "stuck" in pain. I hope that by sharing Elisabeth's struggle, you will experience first hand the mechanisms of getting and staying "stuck" in pain. You will also be able to follow Elisabeth as she gets loose and goes on to create the life of her choice. The second chapter provides another kind of social systems context relevant to the shaping of pain behavior and subsequent disability. The statistics show that those countries who try hardest to help citizens to control, alleviate, avoid pain through access to physicians, medical treatment and sick disability have by far the greatest problem with pain prevalence seen in number of persons disabled due to pain. These costly facts should nudge politicians and health care administrators to take a long hard look at the costs and effects of present approaches to pain. The next four chapters present different components in ACT therapy of pain including the values work, therapeutic relationship, acceptance, defusion and commitment. Underpinning all of these chapters is the functional analysis, which looks somewhat different in the ACT model. When doing a functional analysis with the values context, it becomes clear that coping more successfully with pain is a means to a larger end. The ACT therapist assumes that the client does not want to just be rid of the pain but wants to be rid of the pain, in order to reclaim a vital life. The emphasis in the ACT perspective is not reduction of the problem but rather building repertoire in valued directions. A step-by-step protocol showing how to do a functional analysis for chronic pain is illustrated here.

The second half of the book provides the reader with step-by-step guidelines as how to do the therapy. You will find protocols, actual session transcripts over dialogues illustrating each component of the ACT therapy. In addition to doing therapy with clients, there is also a chapter dedicated to using these same ACT principles in consulting with rehab staff and other psychologists feeling "burned out". From an ACT perspective, care providers and even systems of care providers suffer from the same "problem" that plagues our clients. ACT therapists who have a sense that we are all in the same boat may be better prepared to act with compassion and to act more effectively when they share a sense of the magnitude of the task.

My co-authors, Steve, Kelly and Carmen are giants in the ACT field and have worked very hard with me to get this book together. We have together created a new context. Without their persistence and patience with all of the cultural and language obstacles, it would hardly have been possible. I want to especially thank Steve for his encouragement and sensitivity to me as a woman researcher. His words to me from the start of this project were typical of his support throughout: "Go for it." I would also like to acknowledge the tedious, persistent efforts of Emily Neilan and Camille Hayes at Context Press in helping to prepare this manuscript. When I think of this group, and look at this book now, I associate to the words of Margaret Mead, "Never underestimate what a small number of dedicated people can achieve."

JoAnne Dahl
Uppsala, Sweden
March 2005

Table of Contents

Chapter 1

Elisabeth: Getting Stuck

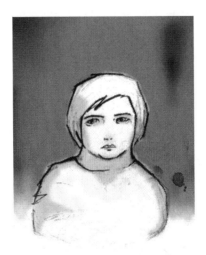

Elisabeth is in many ways typical of an individual who has gotten "stuck" in her pain and stress symptoms and may never return to work. Listen to her story and think about what type of factors might be involved in the process of "getting stuck" in symptoms that result in unnecessary dysfunction and tragic personal losses.

"My name is Elisabeth and I'm 45 years old. I am a childcare worker and I have had the same job at the same place since I was 18 years old. But now I don't work anymore. Right now I feel deserted and disappointed at everyone including you and everyone else who has promised to help me get rid of this pain. Not only do I still have unbearable pain despite enormous efforts to get rid of it, I have also lost my life. Everyone has turned their backs on me which I can somehow understand because I'm not worth much anymore. My employer, my "so-called" friends, the health care system, the insurance system and even my family can't stand me. I guess I'm not a very nice person to be around. The primary care center seems to have blacklisted me because every time I call, for whatever reason, they just put me off. I worry about what would happen if I got a heart attack. They probably would just tell me to calm down and take more painkillers then too. I can tell that my boss doesn't want me back at work. We were at a meeting and I could tell by the look on his face that he thought I was a hopeless case that had cost him a lot of trouble and money when I got sick. Which I can also understand. Who would want me? I never know from one day to the next how my pain will be. Some mornings, I can hardly get out of bed. A person like me just can't have those responsibilities. It was different when I had my health. So I can understand that he wants someone young and healthy to do my job, instead of me. I don't blame him, but it hurts to see that he looked at me that way – like I was useless. I really loved my job and the people I worked with. For most of my life they have been my only social contacts. I lost contact with my best friends years ago. Even if I had gotten tired of doing the same thing for so many years, I really think it was an important job. I helped other women and families so they could work. Children are the most precious things we have. Of course, I miss my job and my work friends. It hurts to even think about it. I really try never to think about it – I pretend it doesn't exist. I usually say to people that I don't care about work, that it isn't important to me anymore, but the truth is, it does matter."

"My family says I am always complaining and they just don't include me anymore in what they are doing. They don't even bring friends home anymore like they used to. I wonder if they are ashamed of me. It wouldn't surprise me. All of their friend's parents are working and healthy. They don't have a chronic illness that means they are handicapped and miserable. I used to bake for the kids and their friends when they came over. We would sit and talk and they would even confide in me. I felt that it meant something for those kids that someone took the time to listen to them. Now, my pain just takes all my energy so I don't have any left over for things like that. The kids understand that when you're sick you just can't go and watch their soccer and hockey matches like I used to. They don't even ask me anymore."

"At this point I can't tolerate any stress at all, feel exhausted, worthless and most of the time, can hardly take care of myself – let alone work, and take care of anyone else. The only small relief I can get from all my symptoms and problems is the pain killer my doctors gives me. You'd think that with all the time I now have on my hands that I could do some of the things I always wanted to do when I was working but never had time. But the strange thing is that the more time I have the less I do. I am much more exhausted now when I do almost nothing than I ever was when I was doing so much more. Maybe this exhaustion and burn out I feel is just a reaction from doing so much before. I was probably really stupid to have spent so much energy taking care of other people. From now on I am going to just think about myself and live so that I don't provoke any stress or pain. I have been on sick leave now for 13 months and have a lot of time to think about how this all happened. Let me tell you about it."

"When I was young I had a dream of being a teacher but somewhere along the line, I gave up those ideas. I was pretty good in school but my family didn't think much of my ideas of getting an education. In the 9th grade I got an offer from the community to go into a one-year course for child-care with a guarantee of a

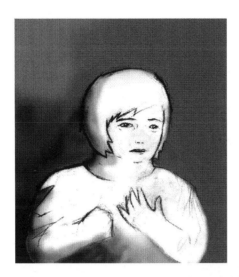

permanent job, instead of finishing high school. Public child-care services were expanding all over the country and workers were in great demand. My family thought this was a good opportunity for me to get a job and I was pretty tired of school so I took it. At the same time I met Eddie who also quit school after 9th grade to start working as a carpenter. His dream was to start his own company as a builder. We got married when we were both 18. We both had jobs and everything seemed positive. Eddie and I dreamed about building our own house and at that time, loans were easy to get and all the costs of the loans were deductible. We borrowed a lot of money and started building our home and at the same time found out I was pregnant with our first child. Due to our economical situation, we had to live in our home as we were building. Now when I look back on it I realize that it was very stressful. Eddie worked day and night, first at his own job and then all his free time trying to finish the house. We soon had three children born all in a row and I had my own full time job. By the time I was 23 we had still not finished building the house. Eddie was working endlessly and complaining of a bad back and I was trying my best to take care of the children, my job, the household and Eddie. I started already then to worry about our finances, the expensive loans we had, and how Eddie was going to manage. Because Eddie worked so hard he never had time to get to know his own children and he lost contact with his friends and family. He also had no time to exercise and take care of himself. When he stopped working he was so tired he just wanted to relax, drink beer and watch TV."

"I also lost some valuable parts of my life during this time. Before I had children and all of my responsibilities I had a lot of fun doing things that I really miss now. I had a group of friends from school that I met regularly. We didn't do anything special but we met every Friday night and shared our life secrets, laughed and just enjoyed being together. That disappeared when I had my second child. There was just no time left over. I also loved to sing in a church choir. I was never a great singer but I loved the quietness of being in church thinking about life. There was no time for doing that anymore when my first child was born. I just couldn't defend doing something that luxurious when everyone needed me. The third really important thing I loved to do was playing soccer in a sports club I used to be in. We played three times a week, had fun and I was in great shape. There was, of course no time for that or any other type of exercise once I started working and had so many responsibilities. When I stopped doing all those things, I lost contact with all my friends. They used to call but I think they have given up on me now. They know how busy I was. I kept thinking that I would make contact later, when things calmed down, but I never did. Even when I did get more time and could have called them I always found excuses not to do it. I don't know why but once I lost contact with all my friends I got shy with people. I wasn't used to being around people any more."

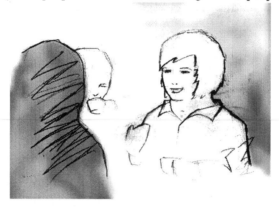

"When we finally managed to get the house finished, we thought everything would be better but instead they got worse. Eddie had frequent problems with his back and he was also periodically unemployed. During these periods when Eddie was home I thought I might get more help with the household and that Eddie might get to know his children better but instead it felt like that I had another child in the house. Eddie was depressed, tired and felt worthless when he wasn't working and he would mostly watch TV and drink beer. He had no contact with his family or old friends either. Eddie needed a lot of reassurance, and support from me. I was naturally very worried about our finances and how we were going to pay off our loans with Eddie on and off work. To ease my mind I took an extra cleaning job 3 evenings a week at the nearby school. About that same time Eddie's mother had a stroke and she needed help with most things. I know that Eddie should have been able to help his own mother but they never had very good contact with each other. She asked for me to help her and I felt that I couldn't let her down."

"During this 10-year period, this is what my day looked like. I got up very early, cleaned up after my family, washed and ironed and got the kids' back packs ready for the day, made breakfast and got everyone off to school and Eddie to work if he was working. If not, I brought Eddie breakfast in bed to cheer him up. Then I cleaned up the kitchen and went off to Eddie's mother, got her up and showered and fixed breakfast, and rushed to the day care center by 8 AM. My duties at work had gotten heavier during these years because we had handicapped children integrated with different functional disabilities who needed to be lifted. I don't know if it was because I had gained weight and was in bad physical shape but it was a strain to lift. My neck and shoulders hurt most of the time and sometimes my back hurt so much I could hardly get out of bed. I knew I should get some exercise, but I had to make priorities."

"At some point I noticed that I was not so cheerful any more at work or even generally and I saw my job more and more as a necessary chore. It wasn't that I didn't think it was important but I really would have liked to try something else. Some of my work-friends took courses and got to work in, for example, special education. I really would have liked to have done that as well. But how could I have taken any courses? Who would have taken care of my family and Eddie's mom? I kept thinking, my time will come ... only it never did. Since I never went took any courses my boss figured I wasn't interested or that I wasn't smart enough so he stopped asking and sent the younger girls. Later when I did have time to further my education, I just didn't have the self-confidence to go. The truth is that I was scared to death of an education."

"On the way home I shopped for my own family and for Eddie's mom, went home, made supper and lunches for the next day while listening and encouraging everyone at home. I would clean up after dinner, help with homework, went back out to my job or parent's meetings, drove back to Eddie's mom to make sure she got

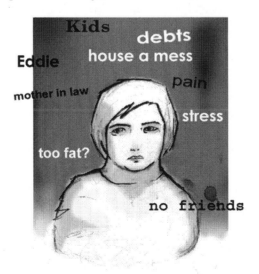

her dinner and put her to bed. I made sure everyone else got food but I rarely made food for myself. Often I would eat fast foods like a hot dog on the way going somewhere or have chocolate in the car. Because I didn't exercise anymore and ate junk food I had gained 45 pounds and didn't feel good about myself at all. Eddie didn't think I was attractive any more either. Our sex life became nonexistent. I told myself, what can you expect after 25 years of marriage, there are more important things in life. But, I wondered what?"

"I felt like a scalded rat running around from place to place trying desperately to meet everyone's needs. But despite the fact that I did my best everyone complained that I should do more and that I was not there enough for them. I got more and more tired, worried and tense. I don't think I was much fun to be around any more. The last straw came when I had come home from work one evening and my youngest son's teacher had called to tell me she was very worried about what was going on with my son. Apparently he had not been at school for the past weeks due to several instances of bullying and fighting with some of the other kids at school. She had heard that he had been seen in town in some older boys who had dropped out of school and who were often in trouble. You can imagine how I felt. There is nothing more important to me than being a good mother for my children. Because I was working so much and not home I didn't know that my son was having serious problems and needed me. What a poor mother I had become. I felt totally worthless. Now I was worried all the time, day and night about what kind of trouble he could be into. I was also worried about our finances and Eddie and his mother and our other children and our future. I couldn't sleep and was constantly tired. My neck, shoulders and back muscles ached and were constantly tense. I felt that I could not go on any longer carrying all this responsibility on my shoulders alone. It was then I called the primary health center to ask for help for the first time. I had never been there before for my own needs. I called first and spoke to the nurse."

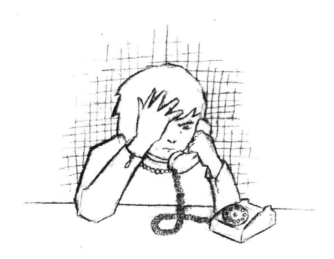

"When the nurse answered, I told her that I just felt I could not go on any more. I didn't know what else to do. The nurse asked me what my symptoms were. I tried to tell her about my worries. I tried to tell her about all my responsibilities and how stressed I was. I told her I had gained weight and wasn't exercising. I really tried to explain everything so she could get a picture but she seemed satisfied just writing down pain in neck and shoulders and gave me a time with the doctor that same week. I was glad to finally get some help. I met the doctor and tried to tell him about my worries and my difficult situation. I told him that I had lost what was important to me and that I knew that the way I was living was unhealthy. I don't think he even heard what I said. He was reading my charts while I was talking to him and seemed relieved to find the symptoms "pain in neck and shoulders" which the nurse had written down. He seemed very stressed and I could see that what I had to say was not important."

"He must have been smart though, because he figured out what was wrong with me very quickly. He pushed hard on different places on my neck and shoulders and some other places that really hurt. I never thought these places hurt more than others but after he pushed on them I started thinking more about them. The doctor said he thought I probably had fibromyalgia and that I could probably use some time off work, two weeks he said to start with and suggested some painkillers I could start using. I never asked for either sick leave or pills but I was relieved to hear that he knew what was wrong with me and how to cure me. He suggested that I also could go to a group meeting for people like me with this diagnosis and gave me a referral to a physical therapist. I hadn't met with any friends for so long and missed meeting people my own age. I had never been to a physical therapist and it seemed very nice to go to someone who was going to take care of me for a change. But mostly I was happy about not having to go back to work but have my almost full paycheck. This break was probably just what I needed to get my life back in order. I had never taken painkillers before but if that's what the doctor thought would help me I was willing to try anything."

"The first two weeks on sick leave were like a paradise for my whole family and me. I finally got some order at home and could clean in the way I like to have my home. I've always been a perfectionist about cleaning. I really like to have good order and a clean house. I wouldn't want people to say that I was a sloppy housekeeper or that my children and Eddie, didn't have clean-ironed clothes. I also got Eddie's mom's apartment in order and even washed the windows. She was very happy to have me around more for company. She has been very lonely since her stroke and I was glad to have more time for her. But mostly my own family was very, very happy to have their mom home full time. I baked like I used to and they came home to the smell of fresh buns after school, and they didn't have to fight over who was going to do chores. I was in a much better mood and had much more time to listen to them. Eddie was happy that I kept him company and could make the family dinner properly and he didn't need to go out at all."

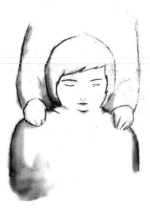

"I followed the doctor's instructions and went to the physical therapist. He was a handsome young man who had very nice hands and listened gently as well. It had been so many years since anyone had touched me or showed me care and attention that I broke down and cried there. He said many of his patients cried when he massaged them and told me not to worry. He always made me feel better even if just for a short time. He also gave me exercises to do, that I never did and lied about because I wanted to go to him anyway. It's too bad that a person has to be sick in order to get care like this."

"I went to the fibromyalgia meeting and that was really nice. I met women like me that had gotten burned out at work like mine. It felt really good to meet others that were in the same situation and could really understand my problems. There was lots of useful information there about the rights of people like us who are sick. There were lists of specialists to see, examinations and drugs you could demand, rehabilitation centers you could go to and even applications for work disability compensation. Most of the people there had been on sick leave for several years and they had a lot of experience of dealing with the health care system, the employers and the national health insurance. I don't think any of them planned on returning to work."

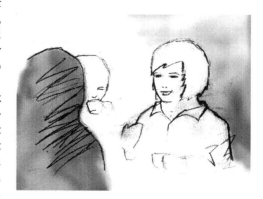

"We always had a lot to talk about. There was a general agreement that it was work and stress that caused this disease we had and that we would have to learn to live with it by avoiding work, taking pain killers and living more carefully.

We also had a course in stress management that taught how to make priorities in order to control feelings of stress. After taking this course I really understood how stupid I had been trying to do so many things. I learned that I should take care of myself and let go other responsibilities go until I felt better. I was slowly accepting the idea of not returning to work. After all, my stressful work was responsible for my pain."

"When I went back to the doctor I knew much more of what to demand and how to say it. I told him I wanted an X-ray to find out what was wrong, stronger medication, sleeping pills, more physical therapy, and that I certainly could not return to work. He said he didn't think the X-ray would show anything more than we already knew but yielded to my demands and put me on sick leave for an extended period while waiting for the X-ray examinations. I had never asserted myself like that before and it felt good to say what I wanted and get results. We had practiced at the fibromyalgia club what to say in order to get what you want. When I told the doctor that I knew he wasn't a pain specialist, and that I could sue him if he didn't give me what I wanted, he yielded."

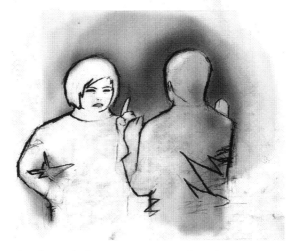

"After a couple of months it was not so great to be at home anymore. Work piled up again at home. Everyone at home actually did less housework than they had done when I was working. They expected me to take care of them and all the household chores since I was always at home. My work friends stopped calling and I knew they had found a good substitute for me who was younger and more positive. I felt jealous and betrayed by them and didn't want to visit there anymore. In fact, even when I thought of my work place I could feel pain and stressful feelings. That really convinced me that work was the cause of my suffering. Otherwise, I did what I was told, to try and get better. I rested, took those painkillers, avoided doing things when I experienced pain but the fact was that I just got more and more tired. That was the strange part, the more I rested and the less I did, the more tired I got. That's when

I started worrying that I might really have a serious disease like cancer or something. If I was doing everything my doctor told me and was only getting worse, I must really have a problem. I found myself worrying most of the time and reading about different illnesses. I couldn't sleep at night and was also worried about our budget – what would happen if neither of us could work. Eddie and I got more irritated with each other at home and fought often blaming each other for the situation we were now in. The painkillers I was taking were less and less effective and I had to take more of them to get the same relief. I even used beer sometimes to wash them down to get a better effect. But the more pills I took the worse the pain became and I was in pain most of the time. I did less and less at home but just felt miserable. I even avoided going out of the house because I knew my neighbors were wondering about why I wasn't working. I told someone that I had a diagnosis but they thought I looked healthy and I could tell she didn't believe I was really sick. I got a neck brace that I started using when I went out to show people that I really was sick."

"Now, 9 months after I went on sick leave I went back to my doctor who had gotten the results of all my examinations and I thought he was going to tell me that I had a very serious disease. But instead he said the opposite. My doctor told me there was nothing wrong with me and that he thought I could go back to work. How could that be?"

In many ways, Elisabeth is a typical patient who has developed and gotten stuck with chronic pain, fatigue, and stress. Elisabeth is far from alone. In the European Union countries, the United States and Australia, persons reporting pain and stress symptoms from muscular-skeletal regions with no clear pathology comprise the largest group of pain patients on long term sick leave. Public health reports (Johansson, Hamberg, Lindgren, & Westman, 1999; Leijon, Hensing, & Alexanderson, 1998; Wolfe, Ross, Andersson, Russel, & Herbert, 1995; Lee, & Powers, 2002) document further that persons such as Elisabeth – middle-aged women working in the public sector – are over-represented in chronic pain and stress diagnoses, sick leave, disability pension, use of painkillers, antidepressants, muscle relaxants and health care utilization. Because of their high medical utilization the societal costs for chronic pain patients are eating substantial chunks of the Gross National Product of many of these countries. But it is the personal tragedies of persons such as Elisabeth who go from active, responsible, and competent lives to that of a passive, incompetent, victim that is the real story of this book. How this process may be analyzed and approached in a way to preserve the dignity and values of human beings is the aim of this book.

Assignment

You will get much more out of this book if you actually take the time to respond to exercises and assignments as you move through this volume. For this beginning chapter the assignment is this: As you think about Elisabeth, begin to identify what factors might be critical to the process of "getting stuck" in chronic pain and stress symptoms.

1) What was the "cause" of Elisabeth's problems
   a) Overload: too many roles
   b) Under stimulated: too few roles
   c) Fibromyalgia
   d) Dysfunctional thought patterns
   e) Other

2) What types of values motivated Elisabeth's care-taking behavior?

3) What dimensions of life did Elisabeth loose?

4) Were Elisabeth's symptoms physical or psychological?
   a) Physical: fibromyalgia
   b) Psychological
   c) Both
   d) Other

5) What were the roles of the health care professionals in the development of Elisabeth's chronic pain process?

6) What have the meetings with health care "taught" Elisabeth about her problems?
   a) The cause
   b) The diagnosis
   c) The solution

7) What had Elisabeth learned from the physical therapist?

8) What had Elisabeth learned from attending the fibromyalgia club?

9) What was the message of stress management: cause and solution?

10) Try and do a behavioral analysis of Elisabeth's problems.
   a) What are the main problems?
   b) What factors are eliciting the problems?
   c) What is reinforcing the problems?
   d) What does Elisabeth believe to be the solution?

11) Do a functional analysis on the following types of treatment strategies offered to Elisabeth: What are the functions of each treatment strategy with respect to short term pain relief and long term effect with respect to activities in Elisabeth's valued directions (does she get closer or further away from where she wants to go?)

a) Pain killers
b) Massage
c) Sick leave
d) Rest
e) Attending the Fibromyalgia groups
f) Talking about her problems
g) Avoiding physical activities

12) Summarize Elisabeth's predicament: what she wants, what she has been doing, what she is afraid of and suggest a treatment that considers all these aspects.

Chapter 2

The Social and Systems Context of Pain

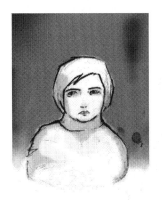

"I had never called the health care center before. I knew pretty much what was wrong. I knew that I had not been eating and sleeping properly and that I worried myself sick most of the time. I also knew I was tired of my job and that I was generally pretty depressed. To be honest, I really didn't think anyone at the health care center could help me out of this trouble I was in, but when I went there, they made everything seem so simple. Deep down, I knew it wasn't as simple as they said but it made everything easier to let them decide and to do as they suggested. Who knows? These people are educated and seem to know what they are talking about. After a while I started believing in this diagnosis and the treatments they were telling me to do. It was easier to take that road than what I was thinking, besides that, there was no other kind of help. What else could I have done? I have been thinking about why it is only women who have the problems I have. At the day care center, we were only women who worked there, it was mostly only the moms who came to get the kids after work. At the fibromyalgia club there were only women and in the newspapers they only write about women with stress and burn out. I really don't believe that it is only women who have pain problems. I don't have to look very far and see that I have a man in my own home with the same type of problems. I think that it is women who complain more and try to do something about it and men just more or less give up. I don't know which is better."

The concept of human suffering is popularly presented in a materialistic paradigm. Popular culture and politicians maintain the idea that the cause of human suffering is the lack of material standards, lack of access to health care, lack of medication, bad working environments, and possibly the lack of free time. Based on this approach it seems obvious that part of the solution to human suffering will entail greater access to free health care and medication, better working environments, better material standard at home and at work and more leisure time. Most of these have factors have dramatically improved in the Western world in the post war era, particularly in Europe. The results of this experience may be something the rest of the world can learn from. They seem far from what the politicians and policy makers were hoping to see.

Why individuals see themselves as sick and/or unable to work and why they seek health care are complicated issues and our attitudes toward pain and suffering are heavily shaped more by our cultures and the political systems we live in. There is no doubt that working conditions and access to good health care are very important factors in the health and welfare of beings. As citizens, we can and do advocate for the rights of workers to be employed in safe and healthy working conditions. But the question dealt with in this chapter is whether these reforms and policies solve the health problems they are said to target, or whether in some cases they exacerbate these very problems. This chapter focuses on the relationship between illness or pain and health-seeking behavior and sick leave; how social and gender issues impact that relationship, and how different health care policies affect health behavior.

Health Care Systems: Dealing with Human Suffering

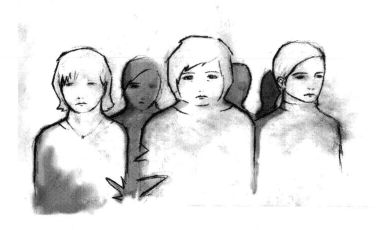

In contrast with the US, all countries within the European community (EU) and Australia have a nationally financed social welfare and health care and insurance system which is expected to meet the needs of all citizens regarding the costs of unemployment, disability, illness, poverty and aging. In principle, all citizens in EU countries today have access to free medical care and free medication. The costs for meeting the national health care needs vary within the EU but are generally higher than comparable costs in the US. Healthcare and welfare service costs in the mid-1990's was 34% of the GNP of the US, but averaged 49% of the GNP within the EU countries and ranged as high as a stunning 64% of the GNP in Sweden (Waddell & Norlund, 2000).

These costs have been rising spectacularly in the late twentieth and early twenty-first century. The rate of expansion for the health and welfare systems in Europe and the US has in effect doubled between 1960 and 1985, but both spending and access to care are higher in the EU than in the US. For example, the number of physicians in the EU per 100,000 citizens is 322 on average, as compared to 93 in the US. The strong belief is that increasing access to the health and welfare system would improve health. Is that belief warranted?

Full Access, Coverage and Free Medical Care are Critical to the Health and Welfare of Human Beings but What are the Dark Sides?

There is little hard evidence that the rapid development of national health insurance in the EU has significantly influenced the general health or suffering of the population living there. Traditional ways of measuring health such as life expectancy, peri-natal and infancy mortality, and deaths due to heart disease and/ or cancer have not significantly improved; the need or costs for the social welfare system have not lessened. On the contrary there is a positive correlation between increased costs in the health care and increased costs of social welfare (Waddell & Norlund, 2000).

These surprising results apply as well to sick leave (or what the Europeans call "sick-listing"). With the expansion of the national insurance system in the EU from 1965 to 1985 the individual obtained much greater freedom to decide about his or her own ability to work due to illness. The effect has been an increasing amount of sick-leave. Between 1985 and 1994 the level of costs due to sick-leave increased 20-30% and early retirement due to illness increased by 15-20 %. (Waddell & Norlund, 2000) In most of the EU countries women show the highest frequency of sick-listing and this gap increases with age (Brage, Nygård, & Tellnes, 1998). Early retirement due to illness increased dramatically from 1980 to 1993 in both Sweden and the UK, nearly doubling in frequency. The three most common diagnoses in work disability and subsequent early retirement are muscular skeletal, cardiovascular and psychological illnesses. In most of the EU countries there was a 20-40% increase in early retirement due to these diagnoses in the early 1990s.

There seems to be a clear relationship between these kinds of statistics and the policies adopted by particularly countries. Within the EU countries the length of time allowed for sick leave and the length of time people are actually on sick leave are highly correlated. Germany, for example, has the lowest frequency of citizens on long-term sick leave and also has the strictest criteria for being sick-listed. The Netherlands has the highest frequency of persons on long-term sick leave and also the most generous criteria, essentially allowing the individual to determine on his/ her own the degree of work disability (Waddell & Norlund, 2000).

The Scandinavian Model

The "Scandinavian model" – characterized by having a strong economy, a unified high living standard for all its citizens and a cradle to grave social welfare and health care system – has been extensively studied for its effects on health (Folkesson, Larsson, & Tegle, 1993; Olson, Hansen, & Eriksson, 1993; Svensson & Brorson, 1997). For example, Sweden spends a larger portion of GNP on health and welfare than any other EU country and at the same time has the greatest number of persons on short and long term sick-leave and early work disability pensions. In 1987, the Swedish government made a policy change in this area that nearly brought the country into bankruptcy. Prior to 1987 employees had their salaries docked for the first day they went on sick leave, but they were paid from the second day forward from national health insurance. With the intention of not punishing employees for being sick from work, the 1987 reform gave employees 90% of their salaries from the first day of sick leave. There was an immediate and drastic increase of sick leave throughout the country. From 1985 to 1990 individual sick-listing increased from 30,000 to 750,000 people in a country with only 8 million citizens. Being on long-term sick leave and/or early disability pension became a new and accepted part of life in Sweden.

Unable to mount the increasingly high costs of this reform, in 1993 the Swedish government reverted back to the original "no pay for the first day sick" policy, and the level of financial reimbursement from national health insurance for sick days was also reduced from 90% to 70% of full salary. These two reforms resulted in an immediate 50% drop of the sick-listing frequency and a significant drop in early retirement.

This decreasing trend in the frequency of sick-listing continued until 1997 when, after government elections, the amount of salary when on sick leave was changed back to 90%. By 2002 the frequency of individuals on short and long-term sick leave was at a record high, costing the Swedish government 15% of the GNP (Rydh, 2002). A government agency report on this increase documented the problem (Rydh, 2002). The diagnoses causing this significant increase in sick leave were chronic pain (particularly muscular skeletal), chronic fatigue and stress related disorders. The greatest increases in prescribed medication during this same time were: painkillers, anti-depressants, lipid lowering drugs and drugs inhibiting gastric acid to prevent ulcers. It is noteworthy that these drugs are sometimes called "lifestyle" drugs since they are used most commonly to correct for problems caused by an unhealthy lifestyle rather than a "medical" problem. The report did not blame the increase on sick-leave policy changes, but on stress in public health working environments due to staff and budget cutbacks.

Like primary care in most Western societies, the heath-care system in Sweden and other countries (for example, Spain) is built to diagnose and alleviate acute and short-term medical problems with relatively simple pathology, adopting treatments focused on symptom alleviation and symptom avoidance. Primary care staff includes for the most part only general or family practitioners and nurses. Patients are seen in quick 10-15 minute visits and physicians see an average of 15-20 patients a day. This means that the physician needs to find out what is wrong and prescribe a treatment in about the time it takes to make a pot of coffee. Difficulties arise because many of the patients who seek help have long-standing pain or stress problems, but these problems will be treated as if they are acute medical pathologies requiring short-term alleviation, not long-standing lifestyle issues requiring psycho-logical expertise. The common diagnosis of chronic musculoskeletal pain is a perfect example. Painkillers, lifestyle drugs, and sick leave certificates are no match for the challenges these patients actually face, but these treatments fit the requirement of a 15 minute visit within a medical model focused on acute conditions.

As a moral matter, all human beings should have access to basic heath care regardless of income level. Still, Sweden example shows quite clearly that human suffering is not eliminated by the expansion of traditional health care services. If anything it appears as that human suffering has increased with the expansion of traditional health care, greater access to physicians, symptom alleviating drugs, more days off, better working places or assess to sick leave. This paradox begins to resolve itself when we examine more closely the content of the health care services we are providing. Our health and welfare systems seem to be built on identifying and solving acute problems with short term alleviation and avoidance of symptoms. The underlying message is that pain, stress, anxiety, or difficulty should not or cannot be part of a meaningful, healthy human life. These messages are mixed with gender role expectations that seem to particularly impact women, who are over-represented in pain populations. A whole set of myths has sprung up around work, pain, and stress. These include:

- If we are not perfectly healthy we should not work.
- Work has become more demanding and stressful than it used to be and that change is the cause of the increases being seen in pain, burn-out and sick leave.
- If work is the cause of pain or stress, the solution is to avoid or rest from work to become well.
- Women are stressed out because they have too many responsibilities and roles to play.
- Women need to learn to make priorities and to say no.

In alignment with these and similar myths, we seem to have created a health-care system and a society that may well create and reinforce ill health, dysfunction, reduced life quality and long-standing symptoms. The greater the degree to which our social and health insurance allows us humans beings to avoid pain and stress generally and specifically in the working situation by means of sick leave, the more we avoid. The more we avoid negative feelings the greater the work absenteeism, life absenteeism and consumption of painkillers, tranquilizers and other drugs. There is an alternative, and it is one with increasing empirical support. We need to adopt a model of human functioning that decreases the impact of negative thoughts or feelings, and increases action that accords with long term behavioral goals. This requires that the structure and organization of primary care be adapted for persons with long-term psychosocial problems. In also requires that we adopt treatment strategies more focused on acceptance, exposure, and values than short-term alleviation and avoidance of difficult private experiences. Instead of myths, we need a health-care model based on hard facts:

- The greater access to physicians and health care adopting a traditional medical model, the greater the help-seeking behavior and the more frequency of illness.
- The more painkillers available, the more pain sensitive we become.
- The more our health care system helps us to avoid unpleasant feelings, the less we tolerate them, the more we believe it is abnormal to have them, and the more we do.
- Persons who avoid the workplace and work-like activities by going on sick leave experience more pain and disability than those who go to work.
- Women do not have more pain and stress than do men but they do seek help more than men.
- Women with multiple roles are healthier and have better life quality than do women with single roles.
- Care-giving based on sound psychological principles enhances health.

Health Care Seeking, Sick-listing Rehabilitation and Return to Work

The relationship between illness, health seeking behavior, inability to work, sick-listing, early retirement and the health care system is complicated. The general model seems to be that a person gets sick, seeks help from medical professionals to get rid of the illness, gets a correct diagnosis, the diagnosis leads to a remedy, the person gets well and returns to work and normal life. If the person doesn't get well due to illness, the proportion of disability is easy to determine and should be applied. None of these beliefs hold true. Health care seeking behavior is often elicited more by discomfort and fear rather than by illness, health care professionals cannot verify the pathology in most cases, a clear diagnosis is often difficult to provide, the typical remedy provided by health care professionals may do more harm than good, and whether the person returns to work or not may have little to do with their symptoms (Robinson & Hayes, 1997; Englund, 2000).

Why Individuals See Themselves as Sick and Seek Health Care

There is very little evidence that disease, health seeking behavior, sick-listing, and perceived work disability are causally related and, in addition, there is little evidence that a physician can make any valid judgment as to an individuals' work capacity (Englund, 2000). Robinson and Hayes (1997) found that health care seeking behavior was determined by discomfort, need for control and confidence in the health care resources not degree of illness. Feelings of discomfort were most likely to stimulate help seeking behavior, but this discomfort was not just current ("My back is starting to hurt again"), it also arose from anticipated negative consequences ("If I don't take that cortisone injection, I won't be able to get out of bed tomorrow"). Individuals vary greatly both in levels of anticipatory concern for discomfort and in their tolerance of it. Most persons feel anxious when they are unable to control mental or physical pain. Persons with little tolerance for pain, discomfort, and the anxiety they can evoke, are more likely to seek help with the aim of reducing all of these unpleasant feelings. Unfortunately, short term alleviation of discomfort does not change this fundamental dynamic. Instead, it can reinforce a low tolerance level for pain, stress and discomfort and increase the control exerted by anticipatory worries about them (Robinson & Hayes, 1997).

These differences help explain why some people feel they are sick and work while others feel they are sick and do not go to work. In a study of pain and stress symptoms and sick leave among health care workers within a county public health system, there was no difference between the frequency or intensity of pain and stress symptoms between those health care workers who were working and those who were on sick leave (Linton & Buer, 1995). Rather, the differences between those who worked and those who were on sick leave had to do with distress tolerance, coping strategies, and beliefs about symptoms. Those persons who were more likely to be on sick leave were those who showed low tolerance for pain and stress, used passive and emotional focused coping strategies, and believed that pain and stress was caused by work. Other studies have shown similar results (e.g., Aronsson, Gustausson & Dallner, 2000).

These facts help show why the traditional medical model approach is so ineffective when faced with the problem of chronic pain and disability: these are very dominantly psychosocial problems. Perceived health status and tolerance for symptoms are far better predictors of work disability than are objective measures of health (Grossi, Soares, Angesleva, & Perski, 1999; Vendrig, 1999). It is how the person reacts to the symptom, rather than the symptom itself that determines health seeking behavior, disability and sick-listing (Saunders, Korff, & Grothaus, 2000; Linton, 2002). The traditional medical model does not target this key variable at all, and, worse, implicitly contains a psychologically unhealthy model of coping and distress tolerance.

Factors Involved in Rehabilitation Following Physical Trauma

There are many studies showing that it is not the physical damage following a trauma, but rather how you react to it that is critical to rehabilitation and return to normal life. The most telling studies of this kind are those related to medically well-specified conditions.

Heart attack is one of the best defined and well known phenomena within medical science. The pathology is fairly well understood, and the damage that occurs during a heart attack can be well specified. Medical evaluation with respect to degree of illness and subsequent work capacity after a heart attack should thus be fairly straightforward in comparison to other more complicated or lesser known illnesses.

Despite that relative clarity, follow up of heart attack patients shows no correlation between physical pathology such as the degree of heart muscle damage, complications following surgery, or work EKG and the rate of return to work or degree of disability in heart attack patients (Riegal, 1993). The factors that correlate with return to work are psychological factors such as worry, the impact of negative emotions and depressive thoughts, and negative beliefs about one's general health. A similar study on the impact of heart attack for men under 60 years of age, showed that returning to work was predicted not by physical pathology but by a higher socio-economic status, a higher rating on internal locus of control (belief that I am responsible for my health) and a lower rating of depressive thoughts following the infarction (Abbott & Berry, 1991).

Similar results have been found in another well-specified medical condition: head injury. In a study of a large group of working age head injury patients, the degree of brain damage as measured by time in coma or brain functioning were poor predictors of rehabilitation time and resulting disability (Melamed, Grosswasser, & Stern, 1992). The best predictor of returning to a normal life including work was the patient's acceptance of the trauma and its resulting impact. Examples of the questions in these instruments were: "if it weren't for my sickness I would be a better person" and "because of my sickness I am almost always miserable."

The same results have been found in spinal cord injury, yet another well-specified traumatic condition. Krause (1992) showed that psychological factors such as acceptance and willingness to take responsibility for one's predicament were more crucial for rehabilitation than the actual damage or degree of functional paralysis.

It is hard to look at the available data without reaching a rather startling conclusion: the severity of a disease has little to do with successful rehabilitation and return to work. It is the psychological factors (reaction to the trauma) rather than the actual degree of damage that is critical for the rehabilitation process following a physical trauma. People facing injury, trauma, or pain need to make psychological adjustments in order to continue functioning. What those adjustments are is the very topic of this book.

How Does the Physician Determine Work Disability?

Several studies have investigated factors that influence the physician's judgment of the patient's work disability. Here too the data point to a pathological interconnection between the psychological processes that lead to chronic pain and disability and the traditional health care system. Controlling for actual symptom level or extent of known injury, physicians tend to judge patients to be unable to work when they: express a high level of disability and worry about their symptoms (Englund, 2000); complain more about symptoms and have a negative expectation about being able to work (Grossi et al., 1999); and believe that symptoms were caused by work and saw work as dangerous (Burton et al., 1997; Linton & Hallden, 1998). In short, physicians reinforce precisely those factors in patient's that predict long-term disability and chronic pain, including worry, distress intolerance, avoidance, fear, inaccurate beliefs about causes of medical problems, and simply wanting to be sick-listed (Englund, 2000). Yielding to these unhealthy psychological processes supports patient's in choices and tendencies that can literally destroy a human life.

Superficially, it is the physician who determines degree of disability and makes decisions about sick leave based on pathological findings. The reality is quite different. Whether or not an individual goes on sick leave is in fact determined by the individual's psychological approach to pain and distress, and how that is expressed to the physician. Those individuals who seek and receive help are not necessarily more ill, but they are clearly less tolerant of negative emotions, more entangled with negative thoughts, and more distressed about their physical symptoms. The medical system provides short-term symptom alleviation at the cost of a pathological cycle of negative reinforcement resulting in more worry, distress, and help-seeking, and an even lower tolerance for discomfort.

Social Factors Influence

From a medical history perspective the phenomena of diffuse pain with no pathology in human beings has been a constant over cultures and time. Historical medical reports show patients seeking help for symptoms nearly identical to what we today call Fibromyalgia (Johannisson, 1997). Only the diagnosis names have changed throughout history: hysterical, hypochondriac, neurasthenic, and neurotic.

Johannisson (1997) suggests that the phenomena of pain can be broken into two eras: Integrated pain, when pain was considered a natural part of human life, and naked pain, when pain was regarded as a neurogenic phenomena belonging to the medical world. Human beings will inevitably get sick, grow old, and have pain, but pain exists only as we experience it. It is not that pain itself has increased – rather our willingness to accept pain that has decreased. Ironically, she suggests that the seed of this shift is treatment itself: *when pain was unavoidable, humans accepted, tolerated, and lived with integrated pain but when pain became avoidable it became naked and unbearable.* There were no very effective medicines to reduce pain in the 16th and 17th century. Opium was used in the beginning of the 18th century in postoperative situations. Laughing gas and chloroform were introduced in the mid 19th century. Morphine was used from the later half of the 19th century followed by cocaine and aspirin at the turn of the 20th century. Novocain was introduced and used by dentists at the beginning of the 20th century. Johannisson suggests that our attitude towards pain changed with the introduction of painkillers. The definition of anesthesia means literally to "not feel." Prior to the 17th century, pain was accepted as an unavoidable part of life. After the introduction of painkillers that made pain avoidable, it became intolerable. This suggests that intolerance of pain is a modern phenomena created by the spread of commercially available painkillers. Our negative reactions to pain are not purely instinctive – they are culturally imposed.

Others who have looked at pain from an medical-social-historic perspective have reached the same conclusion. Allan and Waddell (1989) and Waddell (1991) have shown that the phenomenon of back pain has been constant throughout human history but medical interpretation and treatment have changed dramatically. Ironically co-occurring with the systematic and extensive use of painkillers, sick-listing and providing early disability retirement, has been an enormous increase in reports of back pain and functional disability linked to it. There is no evidence that this dramatic increase is linked to an increase in actual back pathology – the true increase is an increase in intolerance to pain. The health care system and drug companies have created ways for human beings to avoid pain. The popular culture chimes in claiming that our aim in life should be to "feel good" with no pain or stress. The result is an epidemic of functional disability.

The Sick Role

Nachemson and Waddell (2000) describe the "sick role" as a role where there are fewer expectations about what a person is expected to do. When a person defines themselves as "sick" he or she frees themselves from responsibility for the illness and normal obligations, and instead now has the right to special attention and support. A "sick" individual is seemingly not obliged to actively live according to their otherwise normal values such as: working, supporting themselves and family, contributing to the community, exercising, and maintaining a social network or an active sexual relationship. More and more time is spent with the occupation of being sick and less and less time is spent in other life areas.

In a treatise written over 50 years ago, Parsons (1951) attempted to define the social rights and obligations that a sick role entitles. Parsons assumed that having an illness is unwanted and that the individual has no control over it. He stated that a sick person has the right to be free from responsibility for the functional disability, be free from normal social obligations and responsibilities, and have the right to special privileges, attention and support from society. Waddell and co-workers (Waddell, Pilowsky & Bond, 1989) suggest a modified version of the sick role for chronic illness, since Parson's model was built on patients with an acute illness. Individuals with chronic illness have two rights: they are not responsible for the original physical disease or damage and they can reduce social obligations in proportion to the degree of dysfunction. They also have obligations: to accept that sickness is undesirable, to limit dysfunction as far as possible, and to take responsibility for health and functional ability.

The sick role described by Parsons probably best reflects the attitude toward sickness in popular culture. It has been strongly criticized (Klienman, 1988) but it continues to influence our thinking about sickness. In this way of thinking, having chronic pain, would "excuse" a person from living according to his or her *values*. It would "excuse" a person from family, social, work, health and personal responsibilities. Allowing obstacles of pain or illness to block the road towards valued life directions is directly related to chronic dysfunction and loss of life quality.

In sum, the phenomena of chronic stress and pain with resulting work disability and dysfunction appears to be mostly a modern age phenomena created largely by social systems offering avoidance strategies and little else. The social-cultural idea of being excused from the responsibilities of life was built on the assumption that being "sick" was clear-cut, but it is not. Indeed, the more physical technology promises and delivers symptom alleviation, the broader the definition of intolerable discomfort becomes.

Gender Issues: Women are Over-represented Among Those Seeking Help for Long-standing Pain and Stress Symptoms

Around the world women are over-represented among those with chronic pain and stress (Aarflot & Bruusgaard, 1994; Brage, Nygard, & Tellnes 1998; Johansson, Hamberg, Lindgren, & Westman, 1999; Mayou & Sharpe, 1997; Wolfe, Ross, Andersson, Russel, & Herbert, 1995). Women have been found to have the highest frequency of sick leave in all diagnostic categories (Leijon, Hensing, & Alexanderson, 1998). A common explanation about why modern women are suffering from chronic pain and stress disorders to a greater degree than men is the theory of multiple roles. In this view more than one social role (e.g. paid worker and parent) causes stress and ill health because demands compete and conflict with each other and cause excessive overall workload (Stevens & Franks, 1999). According to this way of thinking, women previously had fewer roles and were therefore less stressed. Conversely, modern women are constantly juggling multiple responsibilities and are never fully achieving her goals in any area.

An often-sited study in support of this thesis is that of Lundberg, Mårderg and Frankenhauser (1994) who investigated the differences in psycho-physiological stress responses between men and women. In this study and one that followed (Lundberg, 1996), men and women reacted with differently with respect to levels of stress responses upon coming home from work (women's blood pressure went up and men's went down). This study concluded that the total workload of paid and unpaid work was higher for women than men and that women were generally under higher stress levels than were men. Women tend to be caregivers, both for children and older adults (National Alliance for Caregiving and the American Association for Retired Persons, 1997). The relationship between stress and cardiovascular morbidity and mortality is higher for caregivers as compared to non-caregivers (Kral et al., 1997). Caregivers and non-caregivers show comparable hemodynamic responses in clinical and work settings but caregivers show a significant increase in blood pressure levels relative to non-caregivers following work, especially in the presence of the care recipient. The conclusions are that women are similar to men in general work situations but have increased stress levels in the unpaid caregiving situations after work.

This simple picture has been complicated by more recent evidence on the impact of multiple roles. In contradiction to this reasoning the *enhancement hypothesis* proposes that occupying several social roles provides the individual with a range of sources of positive social interaction, pleasurable activity, achievement and status all of which are related to good health and well being. In a study by Lee and Powers (2002) pain and stress symptoms and health care utilization were investigated among women with different numbers of roles (paid worker, partner, mother, student, family caregiver). Results of this study showed that middle-aged women with three or more roles had significantly better health and well-being than did women with fewer roles. Multiple role occupancy appears to provide both stimulation and satisfaction in women's lives (Park & Liao, 2000). Holding multiple roles has been shown to have positive health effects not only on women themselves, but also on families and communities (Aube, Fleury & Smetana, 2000). Indeed, a lack of social roles has a negative impact on women's health. Dautzenberg, Diederiks, Philipsen and Tan (1999) found that middle age women who occupied no social roles had the highest levels of distress and those women who took upon themselves unusually stressful roles as caregivers actually reduced distress. In a study investigating social roles of retired persons, Moen, Erickson, and Dempster-McClain (2000) showed that an increase of social roles among the elderly in retirement homes as, for example, participating in volunteer work, religious community or political organizations to be related to increase in well-being and health.

Summarizing all of this literature, it appears that women are stressed, stimulated and enhanced by multiple roles. A good balance of different and meaningful roles seems to be positive for good health and well-being for middle-aged and older women. There is also evidence to show that multiple roles are enhanced by a vital social network (Orth-Gomer, 1998; Reifman, Bienat, & Lang, 1991). The problem may not be that women are doing too many different things; *the problem may be that women are not doing enough different and valued things.* Women like Elisabeth may be focusing too much time and energy in caregiving only and ignoring other vital and valued areas. A vital social network, physical exercise, education, quiet time for reflection, development of own interests, a nutritious diet are just examples of what cushions us from developing chronic health problems. Stated another way, it is the breadth, flexibility, and meaningfulness of our roles and behaviors that defines health. Good health does not mean ease.

Conclusion

There are working environments that do cause ill health, and human beings should not have to adapt to a dangerous or unhealthy working environment. Furthermore, we do not put the blame of overuse of sick leave or medication on the individual. But it is very clear that socio-cultural and gender issues dominantly influence what determines health care seeking, sick-listing, recovery and return to normal life and work following illness and long-standing pain. Health care systems, insurance systems, public policy, and the culture at large offer human beings who are suffering an unhealthy menu list of short-term alleviation and avoidance strategies, while more sustaining options are ignored. People are starving for attention to their real needs, while being told to chase the chimera of "feeling good" before real living can begin. Systems which offer avoidance strategies to alleviate human suffering produce a stream of individuals who have fallen into an avoidance trap and – seeing no other alternative – are busy digging themselves into chronic symptoms and personal tragedy.

Assignment

1) Describe your health care system and the types of strategies offered to persons who apply for help with chronic pain or stress.

2) How are the purposes of the strategies used described? For example, are drugs said to be given to relieve pain or sick leave with the aim of lessening stress?

3) What type of function are these strategies likely to have on the symptoms presented?

4) Considering the health care workers themselves, how can the strategies offered by your health care system be described functionally? For example, how do the alternatives offered fit the role of the physicians, nurses, and assistants in the clinic?

5) Consider the physician and other health care workers in your setting and time, information and situation in which patients are seen. Now consider each assessment domain below and possible answers or areas. Which of these areas or answers might there be adequate information or time with the usual patient for the professional to understand or deal with this area:

   a) Why the person has come
      i) Because they are worried about something.
      ii) Because they want an explanation for their symptoms.
      iii) Because they want a diagnosis.
      iv) Because they want a solution.

   b) The symptoms the person presents
      i) A new and temporary symptom.
      ii) A longstanding symptom.
      iii) A symptom with a clear pathological foundation.
      iv) A symptom with an unclear and complicated cause.
      v) A psychosomatic background.

   c) What the person believes the cause to be
      i) A specific pathological cause.
      ii) An accident.
      iii) Work related cause.
      iv) Psychological.

   d) What the person believes the solution to be
      i) Quick relief in the form of drugs to alleviate or reduce the problem.
      ii) Relief from work in the form of sick leave.

          iii) Take away the problem with surgery.
          iv) Other ways of symptom alleviation.
          v) Lifestyle changes.

   e) How person thinks a professional can help them
          i)   Give them an explanation.
          ii) Give them a diagnosis.
          iii) Do examinations or send the client for further investigations.
          iv) Provide symptom alleviation by means of drugs.

   f)   The kinds of solutions that have already tried to alleviate, reduce or manage the problem and how they have worked

6) How could these meetings with the health care system be organized in another way so that symptoms are less likely to be reinforced and maintained in the long run?

Chapter 3

All this Suffering, Pain, and Disability: What is Wrong?

Three Approaches to the Understanding and Treatment of Chronic Pain and Human Suffering

"Some day, there will be a medical breakthrough and researchers will find the cause of pain and cure it."

" I just haven't found the right doctor yet."

"I wish people could see that I was sick so they would know why I can't work."

"I don't dare go out and do things because then people won't think I am really sick."

"The physical therapist told me that the cause of my pain was all the lifting I did at work."

" My life today mostly revolves around taking care of my pain."

"You can read in the newspapers every single day about how people are stressed out at work".

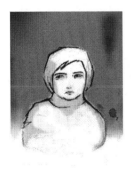 "I am really confused. The doctor gave me a diagnosis and told me what was wrong with me and gave me a prescription of pain-killers and rest to fix things. When I did what he told me, I got worse. I really got worried and called frequently to the health center to tell them that and to get help. I got the feeling that they didn't believe me and tried to put me off. Then I really worried. The physical therapist told me that it was all the lifting I did at work that caused the pain. But when I stopped lifting and rested, I just hurt more. By the time I finally figured out that it was my job and stress that had caused all my problems, they told me I had to go back to work. Things got even stranger. At the rehabilitation center they asked me what activities and movements caused pain and when I showed them they told me to do those things. Everything they said at the rehabilitation center was the opposite of what they said at the primary care center. They wanted me to stop taking my pain-killers, do every kind of activity that causes

pain, and go back to work. They told me that the diagnosis I had wasn't the cause of my pain. Don't these people talk to each other? I am really confused!"

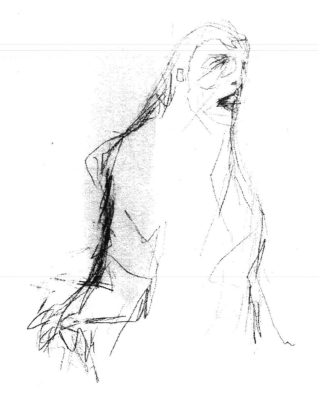

The International Association for the Study of Pain defines pain as follows: "Pain is an unpleasant sensory and emotional experience associated with actual or potential tissue damage, or described in terms of such damage" (pp. 210-211, Merskey & Bogduk, 1994). This definition explicitly affirms that the pain experience has both a sensory and an emotional-evaluative component and acknowledges that pain may occur in the absence of physical pathology.

Pain is one of the most frequent reasons that patient visit a physician and at the same time it is one of the least understood symptoms. Chronic pain is, to a large degree, regarded as acute pain that has persisted. The most common treatments for pain in primary care centers are pain killers, physical therapy, manipulation, and transcutaneous electrical nerve stimulation (TENS). Unfortunately, the scientific evidence supporting the effectiveness of these methods on pain relief or functioning of the patient of the patient is limited (Bigos, Bowyer, Braen et al., 1994). There is a need for new thinking.

In this chapter, three theoretical models of human pain and suffering are presented: medical / pathological; behavior medicine / Cognitive behavior therapy;

and Acceptance and Commitment Therapy. In some ways these three models represent a continuum of development over time with respect to the understanding of human suffering. Even though the models overlap, the difference between them has important consequences with regard to the ways in which we approach the individual who is suffering from chronic pain and stress.

The Medical/Pathological Model of Pain

A common assumption about pain is that it is either somatic ("real") or psychogenic ("not real"). This way of thinking stems from the mechanistic scientific tradition upon which medical science is built. Within this tradition, the body is conceptualized entirely as a collection of biological parts, relations, and forces: as a biomachine. It is assumed that there are defective parts, relations, or forces (that is, a specific biological pathology) that cause particular signs (things the physician can see) and symptoms (things the patient must report) to occur. The medical task is to work backwards from signs and symptoms to identify the underlying pathology, and then to cure the pathology or ameliorate its impact. The traditional medical/pathological approach to chronic illness stems from this tradition (Ogden, 1997).

There are times when this model works quite well. Where it tends to fail are in cases in which a) multiple forms of physical pathology produce common signs and symptoms, b) behavioral history and context interact with physical pathology to produce signs and symptoms, or c) common sources of both kinds (a and b) produce multiple forms of signs and symptoms. When these interactive and multiple determined conditions dominate, there is no one-to-one correlation between physical pathology (e.g., tissue damage) and observed signs and symptoms. As a result, signs and symptoms are no longer a powerful guide to understanding the etiology, function, and course of problems. Unfortunately, pain is an area in which all three of these situations indeed are common and most pain experiences are not at all medically clear.

This lack of clarity is initially difficult to detect, in part because medical terminology itself is based on the model. The International Association of Pain (IASP) classifies pain as nociceptive, neurogenic, or psychogenic. Nociceptive pain is said to be caused by the activation of pain receptors that are in most tissues like the skin, muscles, joints and blood vessels. Pain of this kind might include scrapes, bumps, bruises, burns, cuts, and the like. In can also include more diffuse pain, such as visceral pain (pain related to internal organs), or muscular strains. Neurogenic (also called "neuropathic") pain is said to be caused by problems in the peripheral and central nervous system. This might include such things as the peripheral neuropathy seen in diabetes or alcoholism, or phantom limb pain. In this case the painful stimulation does not arise in pain receptors, but in the nervous system itself. Psychogenic pain is thought to be unusual but is seen in certain psychotic states such as schizophrenic or depressive disorders.

Unfortunately, while these distinctions seem intellectually clear (indeed they are clear in some cases) they imply that most pain symptoms can be traced back either to two pathological aspects of the nervous system or to psychological causes.

That is far from the case. We can illustrate this problem with the relationship between pathological findings and back pain.

Many back pain patients describe nociceptive or neurogenic pain symptoms and also show pathological physical findings such as inflammation, fibrosis in the muscles or disc hernia. In a simple biomechanical model, these pathological findings would explain the back pain symptoms. Unfortunately, these same pathological conditions are found in those without symptoms. When the correlation begins to approach zero, the medical/pathological model is not longer useful in explaining pain experience.

One of the early studies of this kind (Weisel, Tsourmas, Feffer, Citrin, & Patronas, 1984) investigated patients with and without back pain symptoms and found a significant number of positive CAT scans for disc hernia among those patients with no back pain. Similarly, Boden, Davis, Dina, Patronas and Wiesel (1990) showed abnormal magnetic resonance scans of the lumbar spine in patients who had no symptoms at all. As this literature has matured, some of the findings give little wiggle room for a traditional medical approach. For example, Boos, Reider, Schade, Spratt, Semmer and Aebi (1995) not only showed that there was no correlation between pathological findings and back pain symptoms, they found that disc hernia was just as common among patients with no back pain as in patients with back pain. Even extremely dramatic and clear forms of physical pathology are not consistently related to pain experience: spondylosis, respective degenerative changes caused by osteroporosis with fractures, spinal stenosis, bacterial rheumatoid spondylitis, and diseases such as morbus Bechterew are all semi-specific causes of back pain but do not always cause back pain symptoms.

Muscles have long been assumed to play a role in both acute and chronic back pain. Here again, despite extensive research on the topic, no specific pathology has been found (Hides, Richardson, & Jull, 1995; Hides, Richardson, & Jull, 1996; Hides, Stokes, & Saide, 1994). According to a common chiropractic theory, for example, back pain is believed to be caused by the locked facet joints between the vertebrates in the spine, which caused the muscles to contract and become spastic. Anatomic investigations including the use of biopsies and injections have attempted to show a correlation between this pathology and back pain without success (King & Cavanaugh, 1996). Despite 50 years of intensive investigations of biological mechanisms of the back, no findings of clinical relevance have been able to show any specific pathology that could explain either acute or chronic back pain (Carlsson & Nachemson, 2000).

What diagnostic words like neurogenic, nociceptive, neuropathic, psychogenic, real, muscle, or existential pain do is to draw us into a world in which structural distinctions can be used to understand and treat an individual's pain experience. They import the dominant medical/pathological model into our very descriptions of pain itself, and as a result less obvious paths forward are difficult to find. Our objection to this model is more functional that ontological. We are not arguing that pain has no underlying physical pathology. In cases where pain has a specific pathology that can be alleviated, like an abscessed tooth, no one would question that specific medical treatments should be used to address the problem. Furthermore, in cases in which physical pathology does not now explain pain experience, future research may show that some of the problem was simply that our understanding of these processes was too primitive. But that does not alter the fact that pain experience is often much more complex than physical pathology alone, especially when pain is chronic. If that is true even when pathology is clear, we will never find a full solution to pain through understanding of physical pathology. Human beings are not merely biological machines: they are also historical, developmental, languaging creatures, interacting in and with their world. The psychological level of analysis cannot be reduced to biology alone, even though it can be approached in a monistic fashion. This book is about how we react to the pain and stress experience, no matter what the source underlying it happens to be.

In the next section we will briefly review the existing literature on chronic pain and the treatments typically applied to them. Our intention is to document the nature and extent of the problem, and to take a cold, hard look at whether we are currently succeeding in our usual approaches to the alleviation of this form of human suffering.

Common Pain Symptoms With or Without Physical Pathology

"It was important for me to get a diagnosis so I and others around me would know what is wrong"

"When you have a diagnosis you can get the proper treatment".

"The diagnosis of fibromyalgia gave me a kind of identity and made me feel I belonged to a group."

"After feeling confused about what was wrong, everything became much simpler when I got my diagnosis, I know how to behave and what to expect."

"People generally showed me more respect and consideration when I told them my diagnosis."

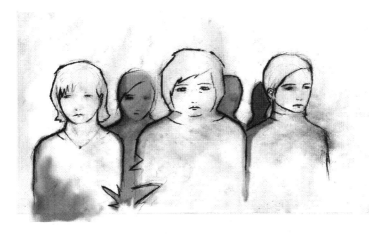

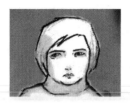 "I felt much better after the doctor gave me the diagnosis of fibromyalgia. I was so confused before that. Everything seemed so complicated. It was much easier when I found out that the cause of my problems was fibromyalgia. It was also easier to tell everyone else what was wrong with me, why I couldn't work or do a lot of other things. Life became much simpler when I knew I was sick."

Fibromyalgia, Neck and Back Pain: The Most Common Benign Chronic Pain Disabilities

Fibromyalgia

Fibromyalgia has had many names throughout medical history: fibrositis, myofaciel syndrome, muscle rheumatism, and many others. Fibromyalgia is classified as a nonmalignant chronic musculoskeletal pain showing symptoms of hyperalgesia (heightened pain sensitivity) in muscles and nearby structures with so called tender points (Bennet, 1999). The pathology for fibromyalgia is not clear, although a wide variety of possible sources have been noted, including growth hormone deficiency (Bennet, Clark, & Walczyk, 1998) and neuroendocrine abnormalities (Clauw, 1997).

Prevalence. The prevalence of fibromyalgia has been shown to be more common in women than man and more common with increasing age. About 23% of persons 70 and older have fibromyalgia (Wolfe, Ross, Andersson, Russell, & Herbert, 1995). Some studies have shown that fibromyalgia peaks at middle age (Andersson, Ejlertsson, Leden, & Rosenberg, 1993).

Treatment. The most common treatments of fibromyalgia are the use of opiate drug therapy, antidepressant drug therapy, anti-inflammatory drugs, physical therapy, acupuncture and rest (Aronson, 1997). The effectiveness of these regimes has been severely criticized by the US Agency for Health Care Policy Research (Bigos, Bowyer, Braen et al., 1994). These treatment therapies are the same as those used for chronic pain in general and will be discussed in more detail later in this chapter.

Neck and back pain. Back pain is typically defined as the state of pain in the neck and back regions with or without shooting sensations out in the extremities. The symptoms are so common that they are considered to be a normal part of life. Nearly everyone will experience neck and back pain in their lifetime. In a medical perspective, neck and back pain is rarely a sign of any serious medical problem (Nachemson & Jonsson, 2000). Disc hernia was first described as a cause of back pain over 70 years ago (Mixter & Barr, 1934). What was then viewed as "damage" we now know typically involves the normal degeneration in these structures. About half of the population has what could be diagnosed as a disc hernia without having reported pain symptoms (Boos et al, 1995; Borenstein, o'Mara, Boden, Lauerman, Jacobson et al., 1998)

Prevalence. Back pain is second only to headache as the most common pain symptom reported in the US. Comprehensive reviews of epidemiological studies in Europe and North America (Andersson, 1997; Raspe, 1993; Skekelle, 1997) show that point prevalence of back pain to be about 15-30% of the population at the time of the interview, 19-43% prevalence during a month's time, and 60-70% prevalence over a life time. In the Nuprin Pain Report (Taylor & Curran, 1985) 56% of the US population reported the experience of back pain at least one day during the past year. Similar prevalence figures have been shown for the UK (Walsh, 1992; Papageorgiou, Croft, Ferry, Jayson & Sliman, 1995) and Belgium (Skovron, Szpalski, Nordin, Melot, & Cukier, 1994). The problem is not limited to adults. Prevalence of back pain among children in Sweden is 26% over a year and 9% at the time of the interview (Brattberg, 1993; 1994). Back pain had been experienced by 12% of the 11 year olds and 50% of the 15 year olds. In a large epidemiological study in Sweden done 1996, pain in the neck, shoulders and back was the most common cause of chronic illness (SCB, 1996). Epidemiological studies show that the prevalence of muscularsketal pain is equally as common among men and women but that women may perceive themselves as in worse health and seek help more frequently (Branthaver, Stein, & Mehran, 1995). Women are more often on sick leave due to back pain (Johansson, 1998).

Work disability and chronic back pain. Only a fraction of these persons with chronic back pain will seek professional help and of those who seek help few will be put on sick leave. Nevertheless, in the US and the EU chronic back pain symptoms appear to be among the most common cause of work disability. What then differentiates those who end up on disability from those who do not? The difference does not depend so much on the amount of pain as on the individual's perception and interpretation of the meaning of the symptom, accessibility to health care, expectations of treatment, and cultural patterns (Waddell, 2000). The judgment of the physician depends more on how the patient expresses his/her suffering than the objective findings. In the often-cited Boeing study, (Bigos, Battie & Spengler, 1991) over 3000 employees were followed during a four-year period to investigate factors that determined reporting of back pain. Besides earlier bouts of back problems, the factors that most predicted back problems were psychosocial. For example, employees who stated that they "almost never" liked their work were two and one half times more likely to report back pain than those who said they "almost always" liked their work. Reports of back pain were not correlated with objective measures of back function and general physical fitness, such as muscle strength, oxygen uptake, height, weight, body mass index, or the spinal channel as measured by ultra sound.

Disability from low back pain appears to be an epidemic that has largely been created by the western health system (Waddell & Waddell, 2000). Disability increases are not due to an increase in the incidence or prevalence of back pain but rather to an increase in the tendency of medical professionals in the health care system to provide patients with sick leave certificates, and to changes in social policy, such as the availability of disability pensions.

Medical treatment of chronic pain at the primary care centers. Next to infectious illness, musculoskeletal pain is most common symptoms seen at primary care centers in EU countries and the USA (Nachemson & Jonsson, 2000) particularly among women (Johansson, 1998; Johansson, Hamberg, Lindgren, & Westman, 1999). A recent meta-analysis examined all of the most common medical treatments given for chronic pain (van Tulder, Goossens, & Nachemson, 2000) and evaluated their effectiveness according to their impact on pain intensity, global improvement, degree of functional improvement, and the likelihood of returning to work. We will review this evidence, treatment by treatment. Rather than refer repeatedly to this source, general statement in the next section can be assumed to refer to it.

Analgesic drug therapy

Randomized controlled studies evaluating the effect of analgesic drug therapy for chronic pain are sorely missing. There was only one study that fulfilled the criteria for a high quality randomized controlled trial (RCT) – it showed diflunisal to be more effective than paracetamol (Hickey, 1982) There are RCT studies of short term effects of analgesic therapy in pain in other areas but not in back pain or general pain.

NSAID (Non-steroid anti-inflammatory Drugs). Six RCT studies of high quality were found evaluating the effectiveness of the use of NSAID injections for chronic pain (Berry, Bloom, & Hamilton, 1982; Hickey, 1982; Matsumo, Kaneda, & Nohara, 1991; Postacchini, Facchini, & Palieri, 1988; Siegmeth & Sieberer, 1978; Videman & Osterman, 1984). There was limited evidence that injections were better than placebo but there were serious side-effects especially among the elderly.

Muscle relaxants/benzodiazepine. There was limited evidence that any of the muscle relaxants evaluated showed even short-term effects on pain relief. Only one study of high quality was found (Arbus, Fajadet, Aubert, Morre, & Goldberger, 1990). In it, tetrazpam showed positive results as compared to a placebo with respect to general improvement and short term improvement in pain intensity. Up to 30% of patients report drowsiness using these drugs.

Antidepressant drugs

One study (Goodkin, Gullion, & Agras, 1990) with high quality and three of low quality were found evaluating antidepressant drugs for treatment of chronic pain. None of the studies showed any statistically significant effect on either back pain or depressive symptoms. Overall there was moderate evidence that antidepressants have no effect on these symptoms.

Epidural steroid injections

Five studies of high quality (Breivik, Hesla, Molnar, & Lind, 1976; Bush & Hillier, 1991; Carette, Leclaire, Marcoux, Morin, & Blaise, 1997; Cuckler, Bernini, Weisel, Booth, Rothm-an, & Pickens, 1985; Serrao, Marks, Morely, & Goodchild, 1999) and two of low quality (Ridley, Kingsley, Gibson, & Grahame, 1988; Rocco, Frank, Kaul, Lipson, & Gallo, 1989) were found which compared steroid injections with placebo injections (boiled salt solutions). The results of these studies were contradictory. Only one of the studies with high quality showed that epidural steroid injections gave short-term pain relief as compared to the placebo. Overall there was moderate evidence that epidural steroid injections have no effect on chronic pain.

Back exercise

Sixteen studies evaluating the effects of back exercise on pain and function were found. Three studies were judged to be of high quality (Deyo, Walsh, Martin, Schoenfeld, Ramamurthy, 1990; Hansen, Skov, Jensen, Kristensen et al., 1993; Manniche, Asmussen, Lauritsen, Vinterberg, & Karbo, 1993; Manniche, Lundberg, Christensen, Bentzen, & Hesselsoe, 1991). Thirteen studies were judged to be of low quality (Bush & Hillier, 1991; Einaggar, Nordin, Sheikhzadeh, Parnianpour, & Kahanovitz, 1991; Frost, Klaber, Moffet, Moser, & Fairbank, 1995; Johansson, 1998; Lindgren, & Westman, 1998; Kendall & Jenkins, 1968; Lindström, Öhlund, Eek, Wallin, Peterson, Fordyce, et al., 1992; Lindström, Öhlund, Eek, Wallin, Peterson, & Nachemsom, 1992; Lindström & Zachrisson, 1970; Manniche, Hesselsoe, Bentzen, Christensen, & Lundberg, 1988; Martin, Rose, Nichols, Russell, & Hughes, 1980; Risch, Norvell, Pollock, Risch, Langer, Fulton, Graves, & Leggett, 1993; Sachs, Ahmad, la Croix, Olimpio, & Heath, 1994; Turner, Clancy, McQuade, & Cardenas, 1984; White, 1966). Of the total number of studies found, equal numbers of investigations showed positive as well as negative results. In nine of the studies, different types of treatment, besides exercise were evaluated such as: physical therapy, thermal therapy and rest. Six of these studies including two of high quality reported positive results and three of low quality reported negative results. The effects of exercise alone were evaluated in nine studies and in six of these no effects on back pain or general chronic pain were found. Overall there is strong evidence for the effects of exercise on back pain but no one treatment can be single out as effective.

Back schools. Eight studies were found evaluating the effect of the common type of rehabilitation programs used for chronic pain (Donchin, Woolf, Kaplan, & Floman, 1990; Herzog, Conway, & Willcox, 1991; Hurri, 1989a; Hurri, 1989b; Klaber, Moffett, Chase, Portek, & Ennis, 1986; Keijsers, Steenbakkers, Meertens, Bouter, & Kok, 1990; Lankhorst, Stadt, van der, Vogelaar, Korst, & van der Prevo, 1983; Postacchini, Facchini, & Palieri, 1988). Only one of these evaluations was found to be of high quality (Hurri, 1989a; Hurri, 1989b) and seven were of low quality. Three of the studies including the one of high quality reported positive results, three reported negative results and in two studies no conclusions could be drawn.

Multidisciplinary pain treatment. Ten studies were found evaluating probably what is seen as the most common treatment of pain today: multidisciplinary pain treatment. Four were judged to be of high quality (Alaranta, Rytökoski, Rissanen, Talo, & Rönnemaa et al., 1994; Harkapaa, Jarvikoski, Mellin, & Hurri, 1989; Harkapaa, Mellin, Jarvikoski, & Hurri, 1990; Lindström, Öhlund, Eek, Wallin, Peterson, Fordyce, et al., 1992; Lindström, Öhlund, Eek, Wallin, Peterson, & Nachemsom, 1992; Mitchell & Carmen, 1994) and six of low quality (Altmaier,

Lehman, Russell, Weinstein, & Feng Kao, 1992; Bendix, Bendix, Labriola, & Boekgaard, 1998; Bendix, Bendix, Vaegter, Lund, Frölund, & Holm, 1996; Loisel, Abenhaim, Durand, Esdaile, & Suissa, 1997; Linton, Bradley, Jensen, & Sundell, 1989; Strong, 1998). Eight of the studies including those of high quality showed positive results in favor of the multidisciplinary treatment as compared to traditional treatment. Overall there is strong evidence for the effectiveness of multidisciplinary programs for improvements in pain experience and function.

Manipulation. Nine studies were found evaluating the effects of manipulation on pain and function. Two studies were high quality (Koes, Bouter, & Mameren, 1993; Koes, Bouter, Mameren, et al., 1992a,b,c; Ongley, Klein, Dorman, Eek, & Hubert, 1987) and seven low quality (Arkuszewski, 1986; Evans, Burke, Lloyd, Roberts, & Roberts, 1978; Gibson, Grahame, Harkness, Woo, Blagrave, & Hills, 1985; Herzog, Conway, & Willcox, 1991; Postacchini, Facchini, & Palieri, 1988; Triano, McGregor, Hondras, & Brennan, 1995; Waagen, Haldeman, Cook, Lopez, & DeBoer, 1986). In five of these studies including one of high quality, positive results were found. It was concluded that there is strong evidence that manipulation is better than placebo for short-term pain relief, but there is no evidence that it has any long-term effects on pain.

EMG biofeedback. Six studies, all judged to be of low quality were found (Asfour, Khlil, Waly, Goldberg, Rosomoff, & Rosomoff, 1990; Bush, Ditto, & Feuerstein, 1985; Donaldson, Romney, Donaldson, & Skubick, 1994; Newton-John, Spence, & Schotte, 1995; Nouwen, 1983; Stuckey, Jacobs, & Goldfarb, 1986;). Five of these showed negative results and one study showed positive results. Overall there was moderate evidence that EMG biofeedback has no effect on chronic pain.

Traction. Two studies of high quality were found, both showing no effects (Beurskens, de Vet, Köke, Lindeman, Regtop, van der Heijden, & Knipschild, 1995; Beurskens, van der Heijden, de Vet, Köke, Lindeman et al., 1995; Heijden, van der Beurskens, Dirx, Bouter, & Lindeman, 1995).

Braces. Only one low quality study (Million, Nilsen, Jayson, & Baker, 1981) was found evaluating the effect of using braces on pain. It resulted in subjective but not objective improvement, and no firm conclusions can be drawn.

TENS. Four studies compared TENS with placebo – three of high quality (Deyo, Walsh, Martin, Schoenfeld, & Ramamurthy, 1990; Marchand, Charest, Chenard, Lavignolle, & Laurencelle, 1993; Moore, & Shurman, 1997) and one of low quality (Lehmann, Russell, & Spratt, 1983; Lehmann, Russell, Spratt, Colby, Liu et al., 1986). Overall there was contradictory evidence making it impossible to draw any current conclusions about the effectiveness of TENS for chronic pain.

Acupuncture. Seven studies were found evaluating the effects of acupuncture on chronic pain all of which were judged to be of low quality (Coan, Wong, Liang Ku, Chong Chan, Wang et al., 1980; Edelist, Gross, & Langer, 1976; Gunn, Milbrandt, Little, & Mason, 1980; Lehmann et al., 1986; MacDonald, MacRae, Master, & Rubin, 1983; Mendelson, Kidson, Loh, Scott, Selwood, & Kranz, 1978; Mendelson, Selwood, Kranz, Loh, Kidson, & Scott, 1983; Molsberger, Winkler, Schneider, &

Mau, 1998). Five showed positive results and two negative results. No firm conclusions could be drawn with respect to the effectiveness of acupuncture on chronic pain.

Summary of the Effects of Conservative Medical Treatment of Chronic Pain

The conclusion one reaches looking at this vast literature is depressing. With just a few exceptions, the evidence for the effectiveness of our most common medical treatments for pain is limited or non-existent. Major scholarly reviews of the existing scientific literature by teams of top experts have provided little support for the most current forms of treatment but this conclusion is nevertheless highly controversial. Indeed, the report by the US Agency for Health Care Policy Research previously mentioned (Bigos et al., 1994) was so controversial among back surgeon's and pain management professionals that The United States Congress eventually renamed the agency, changed its director, and eliminated its previous mandate to issue major scientific reviews and empirically-based practice guidelines in part as a backlash against this report. Apparently many in the medical community leadership felt that it was better to kill the messenger than to listen to the message that a fair and objective look at the state of the current science provides: the treatment regimens offered are most commonly to pain patients are likely to be ineffective.

There are some hopeful signs in the data. The most effective treatment to date is an integrated multidisciplinary treatment regimen. Meta-analyses have confirmed that these programs are up to twice as effective as single-component programs (Flor, Fydrich & Turk, 1992), and are more likely to lead to a return to work (Cutler, Fishbain, Rosomoff, Abdel-Moty, Khalil & Rosomoff, 1994). Multidisciplinary treatment is more of a modality than a specific form of intervention but it suggests that when treatment options expand beyond the traditional medical solutions such as those we have listed above, outcomes sometimes improve. Unfortunately, patients with chronic pain rarely meet a multidisciplinary team (in part because of cost) and the effective components of multidisciplinary teams are still unknown. Much more needs to be done, and it is clear that a full solution will not be found in the traditional medical / pathological approach.

Behavior Medicine: Traditional Cognitive Behavior Therapy Model

Elisabeth: focus in treatment: CBT

Functional analysis: The symptoms of pain and pain behavior are elicited by the work situation, the work place, activities and movements that are work-like and associated with pain. Elisabeth has developed a fear/ avoidance response to many factors that she associates to pain. For example she avoids her work place, going out, lifting, any activity involving arms over her shoulders and any kind of demanding situation which she experiences as stressful. She is spending more time in *passive* coping strategies such as resting, taking pain-killers, seeking help, worrying about her symptoms, talking about her symptoms and reading about her illness. At the same time Elisabeth is spending less time in *active* coping strategies, as she had done previously – for example, exercising, working taking care of her household and garden.

Treatment plan: Elisabeth should increase active coping strategies and decrease passive coping strategies. Through graduated exposure and paired relaxation Elisabeth should be desensitized to those situations, activities or movement which she has been conditioned to believe causes her pain. She should expose herself to work-like situations, activities and movements. The goals of therapy are 1) to return to work, 2) to improve physical fitness, 3) to learn better ergonomic skills, 4) to reduce pain medication and 5) to improve social skills. Homework assignments should include practicing assertiveness skills in her home and with the insurance company

Behavior medicine was first presented in the 1970's as an application of behavior analysis to the treatment of unhealthy long-term symptoms in the genitourinary, gastrointestinal, cardiovascular, musculoskeletal, and nervous and respiratory systems. Treatment for traditionally medical illnesses such as high blood pressure, torticollis, obesity, headache, pain, epilepsy and asthma were developed. At that time, behavioral medicine was applied as a complement to the traditional medical / pathological model. Despite their superficial differences, this integration was not difficult. Behavior therapy interventions are executed at the level of the person/environment interaction, but their traditional aim and focus is quite similar to that of the medical model: control and management of the presenting symptoms.

The first wave of traditional behavior therapy, and the second wave (cognitive-behavior therapy or CBT) that followed both adopted the position that psychological suffering is anomalous, and that psychological health is inversely related to the number and intensity of psychological complaints (Hayes, in press). Instead of the intrusion of some biological malfunction, infectious agent, or toxic insult, behavior therapists posit anomalous, pathogenic learning histories that generate negative thoughts, emotions, memories, bodily states and behavioral predispositions. These are the behavioral equivalents of tumors, viruses, and bacteria that must be excised in order for good psychological health to return. The CBT model of pain includes behavior, physiological and cognitive components that interact with each other. For example, the damage tissue that results from a fall off a horse may influence our thinking about horses and influence how we behave or avoid behaving around horses.

This is clearly a step forward, and the treatment options that this approach opens up are worthwhile. While there are physiological factors that predispose human beings to develop symptoms, such as pain, our best behavioral treatments focused on providing the individual with a new learning history that will reduce pain or pain related behavior in what have been pain-producing contexts. Central in this new learning history is systematic exposure to feared events such as fear of movement or an activity associated with pain. These applications of behavioral medicine are based both on behavioral principles (classical and operant conditioning), and in more recent times on cognitive concepts.

In more traditional behavioral approaches, the goal has been to reinforce productive behavior and to stop the negative reinforcement of avoidance behavior, while at the same time reducing the spread and function of stimuli that elicit pain experience through classical conditioning. Exposure based treatments provide an example. Reinforced exposure to previously avoided situations and movements that patients incorrectly believed to be causing pain is mounted with the goal of improving functioning in such areas as reducing limping, walking longer distances, and lifting heavier weights along with general rehabilitation goals such as better physical fitness and returning to work (Fordyce, 1976).

In CBT approaches the principles and targets of intervention have expanded to include changing negative feelings and thoughts as well more traditional behavioral goals such as reducing passive coping behavior (e.g., taking pills, resting) and increasing active coping behavior (e.g., exercising). There are usually elements of cognitive restructuring such as reframing dysfunctional thoughts, mental training for positive thinking, or the use of mental distraction. Stress management, time management, relaxation training, EMG biofeedback, social skills training, problem solving, activities of daily life training, and reduction of medication may all be included in these pain management programs, along with many other elements.

Through 2000 there were 28 RCT studies which have evaluated CBT as a treatment of chronic pain (Alaranta et al., 1994; Altmaier et al., 1992; Flor & Birbaumer, 1993; Fordyce, Brockway, Bergman, & Spengler, 1986; Haldorsen, Kronholm, Skouen, & Ursin, 1998; Jensen & Bodin, 1998; Jensen, Nygren, & Lundin, 1994; Keller, Ehrhardt-Schmelzer, Herda, Schmid, & Basler, 1997; Kerns, Turk, Holzman, & Rudy, 1986; Lindström, Öhlund, Eek, Wallin, Peterson, Fordyce, et al., 1992; Lindström, Öhlund, Eek, Wallin, Peterson, & Nachemsom, 1992; Linton & Götestam, 1984; Linton, Melin, & Sternlöf, 1985; Moore & Chaney, 1985; Moore, Von Korff, Cherkin, Saunders & Lorig, 2000; Morley, Eccleston, & Williams, 1999; Newton-John, Spence, & Schotte, 1995; Nicholas, Wilson, & Goyen, 1991; Nicholas, Wilson, & Goyen, 1992; Peters & Large, 1990; Puder, 1988; Spence, 1989; Spence, Sharp, Newton-John, & Champion, 1995; Turner, 1996; Turner, Clancy, McQuade, & Cardenas, 1990; Turner & Jensen, 1993; van Tulder, Koes, & Bouter, 1997; Von Korff, Moore, Lorig, Cherkin, Saunders, & Gonzales, 2001; Williams, Richardson & Nicholas, 1966). A recent meta analysis of these data (Linton, 2000) concluded that those groups of patients receiving CBT improved more compared to the waiting list control groups or groups that had participated in other forms of treatment.

Targeted evaluations of CBT programs are difficult, however, since CBT is more of loose collection of targets and procedures than a specific approach. CBT pain programs are nearly always embedded in multidisciplinary programs, which in and of itself are known to be helpful. They include a large number of elements, and the processes of change are not well specified. As Linton noted (2000) these studies failed to show what specific component might be involved in their positive outcomes. This is especially troublesome since CBT is such a broad umbrella that the actual programs in each of these studies are unique, making direct comparisons impossible. Studies vary from a few hours to several weeks; they included out-patients, selected groups, in-patients, and day care patients; both chronic and acute pain was included; and studies tended to be small in size. Furthermore, there is little empirical support for the role of cognitive mechanisms in CBT, so it is not known if CBT is really an advance over traditional behavior therapy without cognitive components. Nevertheless, as compared to the evaluations of the effects of the traditional medical treatments commonly used today with patients with chronic pain, there is significantly stronger evidence for CBT treatment programs.

Acceptance and Commitment Therapy (ACT) Model

Elisabeth: Focus of therapy: ACT

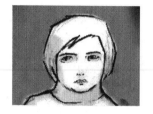

Functional analysis: Elisabeth has learned and now believes that the cause of her problems is a pathological illness and the solution is to avoid the causes of the symptom and the symptoms them-selves. As a result, she has organized her life around her symptoms of pain and stress, and finding ways to avoid or diminish them. In so doing, she is ever more focused on them and struggling with them and paradoxically these symptoms have tended to increase as they become more functionally important. Meanwhile she spends less and less time in activities which give her life meaning. In essence she is waiting for her feelings to change so that her life can start again: she has placed most of her valued actions in life on hold in the service of controlling and reducing her pain. Because of this her life quality has become greatly reduced and her chances of obtaining positive reinforcement are very small.

Treatment plan: The ACT therapist works within a values context helping Elisabeth to re-identify valued directions and intentions. Once this "life compass" is established together with subsequent intentions, motiva-tion for moving towards these directions is in place. Elisabeth learns to become less entangled in her feelings and her thoughts about them, using mindfulness, acceptance, and defusion skills. Exposure to obstacles (pain symptoms, associated stimuli, difficult feelings and thoughts) takes place as Elisabeth moves in the valued directions rather than simulated situations and activities. The functions of the "stories" or reasons given for why she cannot go in those directions are examined in light of her values and goals.

Goals in therapy should be to help Elisabeth move in her own valued life directions by becoming more defused from thoughts and accepting of feelings that function as barriers, and thus increasing the breath and flexibility of ways of reacting to negative feelings and pain while moving towards valued directions.

A major theme put forward in the ACT model (Hayes, Strosahl, & Wilson, 1999; Hayes & Wilson, 1993, 1994; Hayes, Wilson, Gifford, Follette, & Strosahl, 1996; Luciano & Hayes, 2001) is that attempts to control negatively evaluated aspects of experience may, in some contexts, actually increase suffering. In ACT, clients are asked to examine whether attempts at control have had beneficial effects *over the long term*. Instead of alleviating or controlling the "problem" (which is usually conceptualized as the presence of aversive private experience), the client learns in ACT to accept private experiences and focus instead on long-term meaningful goals.

From an ACT perspective the process of allowing symptoms to "get into the drivers seat" is both logical and pathological. Popular culture embraces the notion that positive emotions, cognitions, and bodily states cause good behavior and negative emotions, cognitions, and bodily states cause bad behavior. We expend enormous effort in our schools and workplaces teaching people to feel more confidant, to have higher self-esteem, to be cheerful and optimistic and to avoid pain. From the time we are little children we are taught that we can and should control negative aspects of experience. We are taught that we have the to go through life without pain and stress and that we, in fact should steer clear of these feelings.

From an ACT point of view all of this is quite normal, and indeed is build into human cognition itself. Social institutions that used to resist these processes, particularly spiritual and religious traditions, have been greatly weakened in their ability to restrain what is quite logical. ACT is based on a comprehensive theory of language and cognition called Relational Frame Theory (RFT: Hayes, Barnes-Holmes, & Roche, 2001). There about 70 studies supporting the tenants of RFT, which in its simplest form states that human language is based on the learned ability to arbitrarily relate events. The simplest verbal problem solving situation requires that the person relate words to objects and events ("here is the problem and the objects I have to solve it"), to relate now to then ("if I do this, then that will happen"), and to relate comparatively ("if that happens it would be better than my current situation").

What happens when this repertoire is brought to bear on negative feelings or thoughts? Comparatively and evaluatively, they are undesirable. It is "better" to feel good than bad. Temporally, now can be related to better thens ("I used to feel better than I do now. I need to feel better again in the future"), and action can be taken on this basis ("if I rest more, I will feel better"). From an RFT perspective it is not possible to have a verbal problem solving repertoire without having the ability to focus this repertoire on feelings and thoughts. When one does so, experiential avoidance is the result. Experiential avoidance is the attempt to alter the form, frequency, or situational sensitivity of private events (e.g., thoughts, emotions, memories, bodily sensations), even when attempts to do so cause behavioral harm.

Verbal problem solving strategies work very well with external objects ("if a plant the seeds now I will have food later") which is why the weak, frail creatures called human beings have taken over the planet. These same strategies often work horribly when applied to historically produced private experiences. Verbal rules that specify private events to be avoided generally contain the verbal seeds of these very events. For example, trying deliberately to avoid thoughts of pain is likely to be unsuccessful because the rule being followed will a) remind the person of these very thoughts, and b) may contain memories, worries, or verbalized consequences that are themselves painful. Furthermore, avoiding pain makes pain and possible signs of pain more, not less, behaviorally relevant. In addition, the actions taken to avoid pain may produce patterns of action that are narrow, rigid, and less valued.

Experiential avoidance predicts poorer long-term outcomes in a wide variety of psychological problems (Hayes et al., 1996). Examples include depression (Bruder-Mattson, & Hovanitz, 1990; DeGenova, Patton, Jurich, & MacDermid, 1994), survivors of child sexual abuse (Leitenberg, Greenwald, & Cado, 1992; Polusny & Follette, 1995), other traumatic events (Foa & Riggs, 1995), alcoholism (Cooper, Russell, Skinner, Frone, & Mudar, 1992; Moser & Annis, 1996), and many others. The experimental literature is fairly clear that avoidance and suppression of private events tends to increase their frequency and impact in normal populations as well (Purdon, 1999). Wegner in his studies of thought suppression (e.g., Clark, Ball, & Pape, 1991; Gold & Wegner, 1995; Wegner, Schneider, Carter, & White, 1987; Wegner, Schneider, Knutson, & McMahon, 1991) has shown that attempts to suppress thoughts result in immediate suppression, but later rebound of the thoughts to even higher levels. Higher levels of the aversive thought may set the stage for yet another round of suppression and subsequent rebound. This sort of self-amplifying loop bears striking similarity to the sort of catastrophic thinking that some cognitive interventions seek to stop. Gold and Wegner (1995) calls this an "ironic process"– where attempts to reduce some cognition actually facilitate its propagation.

ACT claims that experiential avoidance is built into the normal functions of essential forms of human language (e.g., problem solving), and is then expanded by cultural forces. If this is true, it requires that less typical functions of human language must be developed, since it would be unwise to attack essential forms of behavior. From an ACT perspective, this is done in five ways: acceptance, defusion, contact with the present moment, self-as-context, and values. These processes have all been extensively discussed in the ACT literature (e.g., Hayes, in press; Hayes & Strosahl, 2004; Strosahl, Hayes, Wilson, & Gifford, 2004; Wilson & Blackledge, 2000; Wilson, Hayes, Gregg, & Zettle, 2001; Wilson & Luciano, 2002), and the basic arguments will not be fully repeated here. We can instead outline the basic approach.

From an ACT perspective, negative cognition, emotion, and bodily states may, but need not, produce bad behavioral outcomes. In ACT the natural experiential avoidance agenda built into human language is challenged on the basis of workability, with the goal of bringing literal language under better contextual control. Instead of avoidance and control, ACT teaches patients how to accept and embrace private experience in the service of chosen values.

Defusion involves learning to see thinking as an ongoing process, and rather than treating its products as a window on reality, to view them as fallible tools to get things done. The same verbal relations that are useful in solving external problems may be unhelpful in "solving" the emotional and cognitive results of our history and current situation. In scores of ways, ACT provides contexts in which language and thought is looked at rather than looked from – in hopes that patients can both use literal language when it is helpful to do so and to simply be mindful of the process when it is not.

Contacting the present moment as a conscious person provides some restraint on the usual process in which thought pulls us into the past or future. Life always occurs here and now. Learning to contact the here and now gives patients a way to begin to let go off the struggle with one's own insides since, like all "problem solving" this struggle is based on the idea that one must be get somewhere else other than here to begin to live.

The most important process of all is values, since values provide the motivation to do change. When a person gets stuck in a chronic symptom such as pain by yielding to the problem and beginning to struggle with it, it is not just that symptoms occupy a larger and larger portion of that person's life – it is that valued and meaningful actions occupy less and less of a portion. As the avoidance agenda grows, the person looses flexibility and life quality and the individual's activities and thoughts become organized around prevention of pain or short-term symptom alleviation. Fighting the symptoms overshadows other valued directions and activities. Like a lighthouse in a storm, values provides a way forward toward a more meaningful and vital life, and helps the person see how far off course experiential avoidance and cognitive fusion has taken them.

The potential cost of avoidance with pain and stress

Medical conditions such as chronic pain and stress fit readily into an experiential avoidance perspective. Because of some of the special properties of language, we avoid thoughts of an aversive event such as pain or stress, very much as we avoid the aversive event itself. For example, if we ask the reader to think about having their teeth drilled, they will likely resist that thought, even though there are no drills present in their environment. Any event related to that thought will also begin to be avoided. If pain and stress are associated with work, work activities or the working place, all of these will tend to be avoided – both in thought and in action. A serious pain problem and diagnosis is not something that is easy to hear or to think about. A permanent pain diagnosis is worse news still. However, an unwillingness to remain mindful of the pain/stress symptoms can have serious consequences. If an individual is unwilling to think about their pain and feelings of stress, consider all of the events that might be associated with these symptoms that would also need to be avoided such as doctors, medication, symptoms, work-events, work activities, and physical movement that precipitate the pain/stress reactions. In principle, all of the procedures that could be used to manage pain and stress will all serve to bring the concept of pain into the psychological present.

If the ACT and RFT view of this process is accurate, what is needed in behavioral medicine is both the procedures that could help the patient to manage their medical condition and skills to cope with psychological reactions to having that condition through values, acceptance, defusion, and contact with the present as a conscious person. That combination is beginning to receive support in other areas of behavioral medicine such as diabetes management (Gregg, 2004). ACT has only recently been used in the analysis and treatment of pain, stress, and coping with challenging medical conditions but the literature here is growing rapidly and is supportive of the ACT model.

We now know that experiential avoidance is one of the most powerful predictors of chronic pain. An ACT measure of experiential avoidance, Acceptance and Action Questionnaire (Hayes, Bissett et al., 2004) was modified to apply to chronic pain (Geiser, 1992), and developed in a series of studies by McCracken and his colleagues (McCracken, 1998; McCracken & Eccleston, 2003; McCracken, Vowles, & Eccleston, 2004). Work with the resulting Chronic Pain Acceptance Questionnaire (CPAQ) shows that there are two primary aspects of the pain acceptance concept: a) willingness to experience pain and b) engaging is important life activities regardless of pain (McCracken et al., 2004). Pain acceptance of pain is associated with reports of lower pain intensity, less pain-related anxiety and avoidance, less depression, less physical and psychosocial disability, more daily uptime, and better work status. A relatively low correlation between acceptance and pain intensity showed that acceptance is not simply a function of having a low level of pain. Acceptance of pain predicts better adjustment on measures of patient function better than perceived pain intensity, and that continues to be true even when pain intensity is factored out.

We also now know that ACT is effective in producing greater behavioral tolerance of acute pain and discomfort. The first study of this kind (Hayes, Bissett, Korn, Zettle, Rosenfarb, Cooper, & Grundt, 1999). showed that a 90 minute training in acceptance drawn from the ACT book (Hayes et al., 1999) produced a greater increase in pain tolerance than either discussions about pain or pain control and distraction training drawn from a popular CBT pain management package. These results have been replicated and extended by Gutiérrez, Luciano, Rodríguez, & Fink (2004) who showed that an ACT acceptance and defusion condition produced greater increases in pain tolerance than a closely matched cognitive-control based condition, especially with high levels of pain. Quite similar results have been shown for tolerance of other forms of discomfort such as that produced by inhaling carbon dioxide enriched air, both in non-clinical (Eifert & Heffner, 2003) and clinical populations (Levitt, Brown, Orsillo, & Barlow, in press). Furthermore, it is also known that these effects depend on the levels of acceptance displayed by individuals (Karekla, Forsyth, & Kelly, in press).

Given these results, it might be expected that ACT will reduce pain and stress in treatment studies targeting these problems. That is turning out to be the case (e.g., Bond & Bunce, 2000; Bond & Hayes, 2002; Dahl, Wilson, & Nilsson, in press; Robinsson & Hayes, 1997). For example, Dahl et al (in press) examined a four hour ACT interventions for pain patients at risk for developing long-term disability from stress and pain symptoms. A small randomized controlled trial show that ACT reduced sick day usage by 91% over the next six months compared to treatment as usual. Multidisciplinary pain programs organized around ACT concepts are beginning to appear and to produce good outcomes (McCracken et al., in press).

From the pathology-oriented perspective described earlier, removal of pathology is supposed to free the individual to pursue whatever life direction they might take. From an ACT perspective, it is more powerful to move toward this behavioral end more directly. The struggle to avoid or reduce pain is not necessary in to that end, indeed this struggle often intensifies the centrality of pain and interferes with a life that is lived persistently in the pursuit of one's values. ACT is aimed squarely at helping clients to relinquish this struggle in order to live a life in pursuit of their most deeply held values. So far this approach is showing promising results. Even surprisingly short ACT interventions (e.g., four hours) can make significant differences in terms of sick listing, health care and medication utilization and quality of life for individuals suffering from chronic stress and pain symptoms.

Moving in this direction requires a major shift in how we think about symptoms and the nature of the problems pain patients face. In a number of currently popular therapies clients are taught to dispute negative thoughts (Beck, Rush, Shaw, & Emery, 1979). Exposure often focuses not on acceptance and response flexibility but on the elimination or reduction of supposedly problematic emotional states, such as anxiety (e.g., Barlow, Craske, Cerny, & Klosko, 1989). Pain patients are often taught attention diversion techniques, like thinking about something else when having pain such as pleasant imagery (Turk & Rudy, 1989). These approaches can be helpful, but so far the comparative studies are consistent in suggesting that an ACT approach is more powerful (e.g., Eifert & Heffner, 2003; Gutiérrez, et al., 2004; Hayes, Bissett et al., 1999; Levitt et al., in press; Masuda, Hayes, Sackett, & Twohig, 2004). More comparative clinical studies are needed before we can say for sure.

The *ultimate* goals of therapy of traditional CBT and ACT for treatment of persons suffering from chronic pain are similar of course. All pain treatment personnel want to see patients return to living a more vital life. The methods of reaching this goal are quite different, however. The ACT model is not yet well known in the pain area, and pursuing this approach requires some guidance.

This book is not a "how to" volume even though a lot of useful information will be provided. The original ACT book (Hayes et al., 1999) and more recent volumes (e.g., Hayes & Strosahl, 2005; Wilson & Luciano, 2002), describe much of the technology in ACT, and book length treatments of the theory on which it is based are available (Hayes et al., 2001). The purpose of this book is to provide linkage between the pain area and these procedures and concepts, so that general ACT and RFT knowledge can be translated into specific ACT programs for pain. For that reason this is not a "stand alone" volume, but it will help open the door to these other resources and to your development as an ACT clinician in this area.

Summary

The aim of this chapter was to present a continuum of three models of pain/ stress analysis and subsequent treatment. The medical model is built on that pain symptoms indicate an underlying pathology, and can be eliminated or ameliorated by targeting that pathology. Traditional behavior therapy and CBT models are built on the idea that pain and stress behaviors indicate an underlying pathological process in the form or undesirable classical and operant conditioning processes, or pathological cognitive processes. Treatment aims at changing associations, contingencies, and cognitions in the service of reducing pain and producing healthy behaviors. ACT is a model built on applied behavior analysis and is unlike the other two models in that it is not focused on symptom management but on changing the function of private events such as pain and thoughts of pain, and on building a more effective repertoire that comports with the person's values. A central theme in ACT is to help the individual to identify valued life directions and start acting in those directions. To those issues we now turn.

Assignment

1) Choose a client (current or past) who is "stuck" in chronic pain or stress and who you know well. Analyzed this case according to each of these three models: Medical, CBT and ACT. Look carefully at areas in which the models overlap and also note carefully what the differences are.

2) Design a treatment regimen using each of these separate treatment models.

Chapter 4

Valuing and Pain

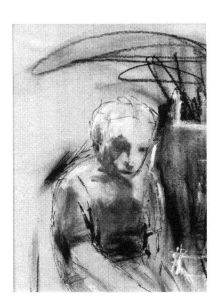

"When the therapist asked me what I wanted my life to stand for, I was completely taken back. It is not a question I had thought about since I was a child. I remember the feeling as a child of being ridiculed when I expressed such dreams. My life has just followed the normal patterns of what everyone thought I should be doing, not as a choice but as the norm. I thought it was better not to think that thought. I was afraid to imagine what I really wanted because I thought it would just lead to disappointment. I thought I had to be realistic and not hope for what I couldn't have. It was painful to answer the therapist's question of what I wanted my life to mean."

Values and Pain

The individual suffering from chronic pain and stress symptoms comes into the therapy office saying "something is wrong, something must be causing this problem and it needs to be fixed." There is a hidden set of values underlying this struggle that when made more evident can make a big difference in therapy.

Taken literally, the client seems to be seeking a pain- and stress-free life. If that was the *only* important direction, however, there are many easier and more certain options than therapy from which to choose, such as drugs, alcohol, or the ultimate avoidance method, suicide. The fact that the client comes to *therapy* wanting relief from symptoms suggests that he or she wants something more out of life than merely nursing pain symptoms. Said in common sense terms, pain reduction is a means, not an end in itself, and thus there are more things at stake than pain relief. That is why the person is still alive and going to therapy rather than leaping off the nearest building.

At first the life that the client values may be hard to distinguish from the struggle with pain because the ability to recognize and move toward valued directions has been impaired by verbal fusion and experiential avoidance, and because the believed means-end relation ("when my pain goes down I can start living again") is so conventional and universally supported as to be invisible. The client suffering from chronic pain, stress, or exhaustion is not without values. By bringing them out into the open they can serve their function of motivating behavior and creating purpose and meaning even in the face of overwhelming symptoms and the enormous difficulties of rehabilitation. Your job as a therapist is to awaken the client's connection to their values. The client's values will be used as the context and compass, which will guide both you and the client in the therapeutic process. In this chapter we will consider the theoretical clinical issues raised by values work and will begin to describe how we assess this area. We will return to the assessment issue in more detail in a later chapter.

Values and Clinical Goals for the Client with Chronic Pain

Using values as the context, the goals of ACT can be described as follows:
1) Defining life directions
2) Separating values from social, family or community pressures
3) Defining life activities consistent with these directions
4) Identifying "hooks," barriers, or obstacles that pull the client off course
5) Teaching methods for diminishing these barriers
6) Fostering larger patterns of effective action linked to chosen values

What Are Values?

We have placed this all important question early in this book and this chapter, but for reasons that will become evident, we can only give a partial answer at this point. Fully understanding valuing from an ACT perspective requires full under-standing of the ACT model more generally. Thus, we will revisit this question later in the book.

Behavior is generally shaped by its consequences and is inherently purposeful. "Operant behavior is the very field of purpose and intention" (Skinner, 1974, p. 55). This means that non-verbal organisms respond to the "future" that they have directly experienced in the past. Due to relational conditioning, however, humans have another source of behavioral regulation available: they can be guided not only by consequences that have directly experienced, but also those that are verbally constructed.

There are different kinds of verbally constructed consequences, including concrete goals and values. Goals are specific desired events: things that can be obtained or not. When goals are achieved they are, in a sense, complete. A job, a house, or a marriage are goals. Their status as goals is revealed by the fact that they are in the service of larger life directions. A job may be obtained to contribute to the well being of those served; a house as a way of creating a supportive and loving home environment; a marriage as a way of supporting and enhancing an intimate, loving, committed relationship.

In ACT, we define values as these very verbally constructed, global, desired and chosen life directions. Values can be instantiated in behavior but never obtained as an object. Contributing to the well being of other is never finished; creating a loving environment for others is never done; building intimate, loving, committed relationships is a never ending task. Furthermore, just as they have no end, values are fully present from the very beginning of the journey. As a person takes the first step toward serving others, that action is part of valuing in that life domain. This is why values are so helpful: there are continuously available qualities of responding that provide a sense of direction, purpose, meaning, and vitality to moment to moment actions, and that also serve to motivate these actions and maintain their coherence and flexibility.

From an individual point of view, valuing is something intensely personal, and in a deep sense of the term, freely chosen. There is a subtlety to this idea that is important for the ACT therapist to understand. In broad terms ACT seeks to reduce the unhelpful aspects of human language that lead to cognitive fusion and experiential avoidance, to situation action in the conscious and present moment, and to link behavioral persistence and change to chosen values. As a system of therapy built on a contextualistic world view, ACT relies on "successful working" as a measure of truth (Hayes, 1993). Truth is not found in correspondence between ways of speaking and events, but in the accomplishment of desired ends. This means that values are foundational in ACT: values provide the very metric against which actions are measured.

One logical implication is that values are choices, not judgments. Judgment involves applying verbal metrics to alternative courses of actions. It is illogical to do this with values since applying a metric requires the a priori existence of a metric, and values themselves are the metric. If values are to be evaluated, by what set of values will we do so?

Choices are simply selections among alternative courses of actions. Without language all selections among alternative courses of actions are choices; however, since human beings are extremely verbal, when a choice is confronted there tend to be concurrent verbal "reasons" for action (i.e., verbal formulations of cause and effect). If the selection among alternative courses of actions is linked to, justified by, and explained in terms of these reasons, then the selection is a judgment. If the person notes the presences of any verbal stories, verbal pros and cons, and so on, but still "simply selects" a course of action with these reasons and yet not *for* these reasons, we are speaking of a choice. In that special sense, values are a choice. The distinction is important in ACT because values are the basis of evaluation and they themselves must therefore not be fully determined by literal evaluation. Said in another way, values require cognitive defusion.

The language of "free choice" is a clinically useful language that helps maintain defusion. Within science itself defusion has little role, and the language of freedom is no longer helpful. Thus it is a mistake to *believe* an ACT analysis of values when one has their science hat on. From a scientific point of view, the vast majority of current values are supported by the culture and are hardly arbitrary. Skinner argued that values were present because they contributed to the survival of the culture, in the context of survival of the species (1974), but it is more technically correct to say that what survives is the cultural practice and the gene not the culture or species, since both are constantly evolving (Dawkins, 1982). Practices that are self-limiting (such as universal celibacy or mass suicide) tend not to survive because their ability to replicate (biologically or culturally) is reduced; conversely, practices must replicate to be part of cultures over the long term. For that reason, the values that exist now tend to be broadly similar for most human beings and to be powerful sources of behavioral regulation. The verbal construction of goals and values, and the actions that will produce them, help guide human beings in taking action even when the consequences are remote and subtle. Human beings are able to see and work toward "long term" goals even in the presence of difficulties. Because of their role within human cultures many values are related to well-being at the level of the family, society, and species, not just the individual, and thus they tend to be a kind of verbal glue that binds human beings together.

The fact that valuing is a cultural practice and that, from the outside, values are determined (e.g., by survival of the practice or gene) does not mean that we can substitute this scientific understanding for valuing as a choice in ourselves or our clients. From the inside, values are simply chosen without verbal defense. This feature is necessary for their motivational effects. Just as a science of contingency-shaped behavior does not mean that shaped behaviors are now rule-governed, so too a science of values does not change the nature of valuing itself.

It is also worth noting that, from the inside at least, values are not merely social conventions. "Going through the motions" in values work to please the therapist, parents, or others is yet another form of judgment, not a choice. Thus, values are personal. For that reason in ACT no "correct" list of values can be generated . . . by definition, it is up to each person to write their own list.

Putting Values Work First

Values work sometimes comes early in ACT and sometimes it does not. There are as yet no data on which approach works best with which clients, but in several populations (e.g., substance abusers, psychotic patients) the motivational aspects are so important that most ACT practitioners put a significant amount of values work first. We recommend this course of action for chronic pain patients.

There are advantages and disadvantages of doing so. One big advantage is that all other aspects of the treatment now can be harnessed to individual values, which greatly enhances the therapeutic alliance and makes all of the rest of the ACT work more directly and obviously relevant to individual needs. For example, the need for acceptance and defusion becomes more obvious to the patient when they are applied to barriers that come up in context of seeking out valued ends. The disadvantage is that early on the patient does not have all of the skills needed to make choices rather than logical judgments – thus values work done early tends to need to be revisited several times as more elements of the ACT model are put into place.

Valued Dimensions Used in ACT

It is clinically helpful to examine values in a variety of life domains, since individuals vary in the importance of particular domains in given circumstances or at given stages of life. There is no ultimate or complete list of such domains, and clinicians should feel free to expand or contract the list based on the purposes of intervention, but at least ten have been regularly used in ACT.

1. Family relations: (parents and siblings) How do you want these relations to be? Describe the sort of person you would like to be in these relationships.
2. Parenting: Describe the kind of parent you would like to be. What kind of relationship would you like to have with your child?
3. Intimate/Partner/Marriage relationships: How would you like this relationship to look like and how would you like to be in this relationship?

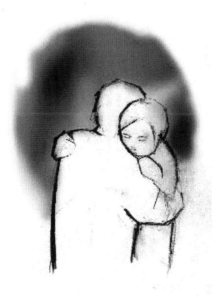

4. Employment/career: What type of work would you like to do? What would your ideal working situation look like? What type of employee would you like to be?

5. Education/personal growth and development: What type of education would you like to have or get? How would you see the concept of personal growth throughout your whole life?

6. Leisure time: How do you see the space for you free-time activities? What would you be doing? Think of your own interests.

7. Spirituality: Describe the role of spirituality in your life. This would not necessarily mean any organized religion, but perhaps the time you take for yourself to find peace, quiet, and perspective on life.

8. Citizenship/community work: Describe how you see yourself contributing to the community where you live and work. This could be volunteer work or simply spontaneous help to neighboring families.

9. Social network/friends: Describe what it means to you to be a good friend. What is it that you want to have in a group of friends? How would those relationships among friends be if they were as you want them to be?

10. Health/physical well-being: How do you want your health do be? How do you see yourself maintaining your health? Describe your optimum level of health for activities such as eating habits, exercise and sleep.

Values as a Compass

When applying the ACT model to chronic pain, we have found it helpful to describe values using a physical metaphor we call the "life compass" (see Figure 4.1). Clients easily relate to the idea of life as a circle containing many different potential directions. When going forward clients know they are moving in a valued direction by the experienced qualities of valued actions. While there is no precise language for this sense, clients use such terms as "aliveness," "vitality," "growth," or "meaningfulness" to refer to this quality.

The metaphor of a compass helps focus the client on maintaining a balance of valued directions. There is no *a priori* rule that all directions *must* be important, but in fact most clients do have important values in each domain. If that is so, it is important to maintain a broad focus. If a person values intimate relationships and friends, spending the vast majority of time working produces an imbalance that shows up readily on the compass. In using the compass we ask patients to try to put something down in each domain. We help refine these statements, distinguishing concrete goals from values, and trying to detect social approval strategies masquerading as values. After this is refined we consider barriers to progress in each direction, which usually involved pain or other aversive private events. This then sets up future acceptance and defusion work.

In our experience, the vast majority of chronic patients are experiencing the side effects of what can be thought of as a values illness. Values illness can include failing to acknowledge ones own values, failing to maintain a proper focus on important values, serious imbalances between values, and chronically emphasizing behaviors that are out of contact with or even at odds with values. Values problems of these kinds are often the underlying "cause" of getting stuck in chronic problems. The individual with chronic pain or stress symptoms is likely to put a valued life on hold while waiting for the internal struggle to be won; they may show a significant imbalance where most time and activity is spent preventing and managing the symptoms, and little time is spent on other valued directions. Since those other directions are sources of meaning, vitality, and purpose, a sense of meaninglessness and emptiness results. Life narrows.

Acknowledging the depth and breadth of one's own values tends to broaden and enrich life. Research examining the link between the number of social roles one plays and health (Lee & Powers, 2002) shows that people who are actively involved in different areas of life, including volunteering to help others, experience less stress and pain than those with fewer social roles. It seems that the narrower our repertoire is the more vulnerable we are to ill health and depression. Homes for the elderly provide a good example (Lee & Powers, 2002). These institutions are normally segregated from society at large, and thus they tend to restrict the range of residents' activities. It was shown that the older retired persons who continued to volunteer in the community and actively take responsibility for social issues experienced less stress and pain than did those who were less active. This implies that feelings of stress and pain could be a signal that we need to be more active in different life dimensions, not cut back. The feelings of tiredness and pain may indicate not that we need to withdraw but that our behavior is too circumscribed and we are restricting our activities to too few dimensions.

Clinical Issues Raised by Values

Values raise a number of clinical issues that may need to be addressed. Not every case will contact every one of these issues, and they emerge in many different sequences.

Absence of Values

The typical client with chronic pain and stress symptoms may tell you that all they want is to learn to manage pain and stress symptoms. They may say that nothing else matters.

To understand this, it is important to examine the learning history of the person who makes this statement. The struggle with chronic pain has often been intense and lengthy. As the struggle pulls the patient into more and more desperate circumstances, the experienced diminishment of life tends to increase the very struggle that is causing this downward spiral. The *means* of stress and pain reduction becomes more important as the hidden *end* (living life) slips away. Ultimately a chronic pain patient is like a person with oxygen cut off – the *only* thing that seems to matter is the alleviation of pain. In the case of absence of oxygen, this is true: without it all else is quickly meaningless. The chronic pain patient is living inside a verbal illusion in which pain is playing an unnecessarily central role in the client's life.

Sometimes patient histories have longer and more complex features that relate to an apparent absence of values. It is not uncommon to find histories of sexual, physical, or emotional abuse in clients with chronic pain (Hamberg, Johannsson, Lindgren, & Westman, 1997). Under conditions of abuse or neglect, expressing values about desired directions would likely lead to disappointment and pain. Just surviving on a day-to-day basis has a higher priority than realizing one's potential.

Furthermore, many clients with chronic pain have great difficulty expressing their values simply due to the fact that they have never been asked, "what is it you want?" Answering, "I don't know" or "It doesn't matter" to that question is likely just an avoidance strategy. It hurts to care about something and it feels vulnerable to share this with others. This is particularly true when caring has led to pain or ridicule in the past.

You the therapist need to be patient in these cases and look at the function of such avoidant statements. You can assume that your client cares about some things – indeed if that were not true it is hard to see why patients would struggle so. Your job is to help bring these values to the surface. This process may take some time as you work through language-based barriers with the client, but the reward will be a lighthouse in therapy for both your client and yourself. The goal long term goal of ACT is helping the client live more consistently with his or her own values.

Is Everyone Capable of Valuing?

All verbal human beings are capable of valuing, and for a simple reason: the relational frames involved in valuing are present in very young normal children. At the point at which it is possible to work toward verbally stated goals, it is possible to value. No one involved in verbal psychotherapy has verbal repertoires so deficient that valuing is impossible.

Indeed, protestations to the contrary only emerge with a great deal of verbal ability. For that reason, it is often easier to identify values among people who are less verbally sophisticated. When clients claim they are incapable of valuing they are typically engaging is a verbal game designed to avoid choice or to avoid the pain of the contradiction between current patterns of living and values. Sometimes this occurs because the client is entangled with verbal analysis and reason giving. Verbally oriented human beings tend to justify what they are doing by giving reasons that fit into mainstream culture. It can be frightening to make personal, undefended choices.

Examination of values in various domains commonly leads some clients to feel that a number of the dimensions presented are not applicable to them. This can complicate the values identification process. It helps to orient the client in a broad way toward these dimensions. For example, asking about parenting can lead some clients to deny that they have any values in this area simply because they have not yet started families, or because they have chosen not to have children. But parenting can refer to a much broader range of issue that include all nurturing adult-child relationships, now and in the future. This dimension does seem to be of relevance to most people. Some young people see themselves as wanting to become parents later: the dimension may be abstract for those clients, but it exists nonetheless. Others may choose to have roles with nieces, nephews, young people in clubs or organizations (e.g., the Girl Scouts, sports leagues), and so on. It could mean that an individual chooses to take responsibility for helping a child in the neighborhood learn to ride a bike or do her math. It could mean caring about the needs of poor children in other countries through charitable contributions. Interpreted broadly, virtually all clients in fact do value some things and not others in each of the domains listed above.

Feelings and Values

We all have days when we wake up in the morning and don't feel like going to work, but we choose to go anyway. We exercise because we know it is healthy for us in the long run, even though we may dread the trip to the gym. Making a commitment in accordance to one's values is one thing, but feelings are not under the same voluntary control. Early in values work it is often the conflict between actions and feelings that comes to the fore. The emergence of "buts" is a classic sign. Etymologically "but" means "be out" – it is an indication that two things are being held to be in conflict. From the client with chronic pain we often hear "I want to work BUT I can't because of my pain" or "I want to be in shape BUT I can't because of my pain" or "I want to have a stimulating job BUT I can't because I can't tolerate stress." In these cases, the client has a value and is aware that following it will likely evoke a feeling. The language of conflict is disguising a more basic fact: The client is allowing the feeling to get into the driver's seat, in accordance with popular beliefs that pain and stress prohibit effective actions. The goal of ACT in these cases is to help the client value what they value (e.g., working) even when they have feelings (e.g., pain or feeling stressed) that are said to contradict (but in fact *co-exist* with) these values. ACT focuses on valuing as an action rather than a feeling. It is by far easier and more effective to focus therapy on what can be directly regulated (overt behavior) rather than events that cannot readily be controlled (feelings, thoughts). For the client with chronic pain and stress this would imply that the goals of therapy would focus on choosing activities consistent with desired directions, rather than choosing to manage feelings of pain and stress.

Values as Choices

The client who is stuck in pain or stress symptoms often perceives him/herself as not having any choices. Certain verbal rules reinforce this feeling of being trapped. The rule: I want to work BUT I have pain or feel burned out, means that until I get rid of the pain and stress, I cannot work. In other words, the client is expressing here a judgment of the situation – a verbal formulation of cause and effects. Essentially, the client is making the judgment that the pain or feelings of stress are causing an inability to work.

The power of values come from their nature: Values are choices, not judgments. By holding fast to this realization you can avoid several common clinic dead ends with chronic pain and stress. One is the tendency to diminish values on the grounds of apparent likelihood of success (as is values are mere goals, not life directions). For example when asked: "how important is education and personal development for you?" the client may say that it is not particularly important because a judgment is being made that this is not a realistic choice due to her life circumstances. As a result, things that the client holds as important are said not to be important, which undermines the role values can play in life. Typically, we do not know how far in life we can go in any given direction. That is not what is being asked during values work in ACT. What is being asked is what the direction itself should be if it were a free choice.

Using values as a choice also helps you the therapist not get entangled in the content of the client's life story. All too often, the therapist gets "hooked" by the "stories" justifying why the client has ended up where she is. If the therapist can stay out of the content of the client's story and help the client simply to make choices in accordance with valued directions, therapy will move forward. Ask the client, "if intentions had feet, where would they go?" As a behavior, valuing is very powerful. Even when the client feels powerless, values and choice are possible since behavior itself is possible.

Valuing as a Commitment

Commitments are only possible when they are based on chosen values. If we make important commitments based on judgments or feelings, whatever elements are contained in the reason are now seemingly responsible fore the alternative selected. As a result, such commitments tend to be short-lived. Consider the difference between a person choosing to marry based on the value of an intimate, stable relationship with the partner, and one marrying based on the judgment that it will lead to financial security because the partner has a good job. If the partner in the judgment-based marriage loses the job, the "commitment" seemingly must now change as well. In contrast, the marriage based on values of intimacy and stability will show flexibly in dealing with the job loss. Commitments based on chosen values are more resilient to changes in life circumstances.

Experiential Avoidance and Values

The client with chronic pain or stress symptoms is often stuck in the belief that they must first manage their pain and stress before they can begin to live a meaningful life. Clients can become so focused on their symptoms that they forget to live. They constantly monitor degrees of pain, headaches, feelings of stress, or how successfully their painkiller worked. In some instances, clients become so focused on minimizing pain and stress that experiential avoidance becomes habitual. Focusing on short-term pain relief may prevent these clients from engaging in valued activities, and thus their quality of life will suffer. Almost before they realize it, clients become stuck in a pattern of deferring living in order to micromanage their pain symptoms.

Avoiding pain and stress is something we all do to some degree throughout life. There is no inherent reason to expose oneself to pain or stressful events. However, experiencing pain and stress are an inevitable part of life. As a child develops and learns, pain and stress will occur. Children can't learn to walk without falling or ride a bike without loosing balance, just as adults can't build intimate relationships without risking (and probably experiencing) disappointment or even a broken heart. Each new experience requires risking failure and pain. The reasons why human beings risk the pain and stress of new experiences is that they find value in going forward in developing their life's various dimensions. There is nothing wrong with avoiding stressful experiences that offer limited opportunity for growth. However, problems occur when avoiding experiences becomes a given regardless of the values at stake.

This is what we see in individuals who systematically avoid pain and stress. Normally, we as human beings are willing to take risks of pain, stress and failure if it serves our values. For example, we may tolerate the discomfort of exercising in service of the higher value of better health. We may be willing to expose ourselves to the discomfort of nicotine abstinence in order to quit smoking in order to live longer. Most of us are willing to risk failure and rejection when we apply for a new job or start a new relationship. In these cases, we are willing to experience pain and stress because we are giving ourselves a chance to obtain something we value. We are never guaranteed success when we embark upon these risk-taking ventures, but are willing to do so because we value some outcome associated with them. It can be said that personal values motivate us, as human beings, to move us forward in life. When we let our values guide our life direction, we find that we are sometimes willing to suffer pain. Values can be seen as a context within which exposure to pain and stress become meaningful.

Recent experimental preparations, following Guiteirrez et al., (2004), have shown that most of the subjects in the condition where pain is coordinated with valued actions, were able to go to the pain exposure for the maximum number of times permitted in the experiment even with a report of 90-100 of discomfort. Contrarily, in the condition where pain was established as against valued actions, the impact on pain tolerance was minimum as it was a control condition without any relation between pain and valued actions (Paez, Luciano, Gutierrez, & Rodriguez, 2005).

Values as the Arena

Listening to and understanding the values of the client is the basis of the therapeutic relationship, as well as the arena in which therapy takes place. As the therapist, your client may share dreams and aspirations with you that they have never revealed to anyone. Clients who are stuck in pain and stress symptoms often suppress their dreams and values, and it can be an emotional experience just to describe them. It can be painful to identify values if the client has made the judgment that they are not realistic, just as it can be painful for clients to see how far away they are from reaching their dreams. In ACT, when clients discover that there are

discrepancies between their stated values and actual activities, the moment is used
as a motivator for behavior change.

By way of illustration, the following are examples of what two different therapy
sessions might look like; one is based on an ACT approach and uses values as the
context for therapy, the other does not. The example is of a 32 year old man named
Bill with longstanding lower back pain.

Traditional approach

Therapist: Bill, as I understand it you have had back pain for a long time
and that has caused you to go on disability.

Bill: That's right. I can't work, I've gained weight because I can't exercise
and I have to rest a lot. I get bored so I eat instead. I just can't seem
to get going and do anything. That fitness test I took here showed I was
in poor condition.

Therapist: OK, you are saying that besides your back pain, you have this
problem with your weight, your physical fitness test was poor, and you
are lying down a lot and eating more than you should.

Bill: That's right; I don't know what to do. I'd get back in shape if it weren't
for this pain.

Therapist: In this program we talk about coping skills. Resting, taking pills,
not working and eating are what we would call passive coping skills.
That means that you deal with your pain by doing things that only have
a short-term effect and in the long term you get in worse shape.

Bill: That's what has happened. But what else can I do when I have this
terrible pain?

Therapist: Active coping skills are ways to manage pain that help you in
the long run but they may be more painful in the short run.

Bill: What do you mean? Will this program be painful?

Therapist: Yes, but it will help. For example, I see that you are stiff and
that you avoid bending over.

Bill: Yes, because bending makes the pain worse. I don't want to end up
lying in bed all the time. When I wear this brace and don't bend I have
some control.

Therapist: We have a program here that we called graduated training that
will help you be able to bend over again.

Bill: You don't understand. I just told you bending causes terrible back pain.

Therapist: If you do these exercises, it may hurt somewhat but you will get
better in the long run. We have experience at this clinic with back pain
and we know that this program has been successful in making bending
over easier. In this graduated training we measure how far you can bend
today and we set up a goal for how far you should be able to bend by
the end of the program. So, say you can bend 2 cm right now and the
goal is to bend 100 cm. You would get a chart and we would figure out
how many cm you would need to exercise in bending each day to reach

that goal in 4 weeks. By following this chart you could see your progress, and that usually helps patients move toward their goals even if it is painful.

Bill: That sounds difficult, but I guess I have no choice.

ACT

Therapist: Bill, Why have you come here?

Bill: I have this terrible back pain; I don't know what to do. I can't work, I've gained weight because I can't exercise, and I have to rest a lot. I get bored so I eat instead. I just can't seem to get going and do anything. That fitness test I took here showed I was in poor condition.

Therapist: How do you think I could help you Bill?

Bill: I don't know. Maybe you could help me manage this pain so I could get back to work and start living again.

Therapist: I get the sense that you want more out of your life than what you have now, that your pain is squeezing the life out of you.

Bill: I don't have a life any more. All I have is my pain.

Therapist: Let's look at your life, Bill, and what it is you want. Where do you want to go? I want to know what your goals are and what's keeping you from reaching them.

Bill: What I want is my life back. But I don't even want to think about that because I know that can't happen because of my bad back.

Therapist: I am not asking you what is possible, Bill, I'm just asking what you want. Let's look at ten life dimensions that are about the same for all human beings and see how important they are to you and what you want in each one.

Bill: I don't see how that will help me with my back, but OK.
(Bill goes through all ten dimensions, rates their importance, writes a sentence of intention for each, and rates how much of his time he has invested in each area.)

Therapist: If you see these different life dimensions as valued directions in life, what would you say about how your life looks now?

Bill: It looks like I got way off course somewhere along the line, and that my life is headed somewhere I don't want to go. And it is all due to this pain.

Therapist: Where do you want to go Bill?

Bill: If I could just get rid of this pain, I would know where to go. I would move in all these directions and live the way I want.

Therapist: I want to hear more about what you want Bill, and what you are afraid of.

Comments on these two dialogues:

In both of the two models shown here, the goals are similar and the component of exposure to pain is central, but the means of getting there are different. In the traditional model where values are not emphasized, the client is motivated through the use of instructions and structured programs designed to alter behavioral functions. In the ACT model, the client is motivated by the value of his own desired life directions.

In the traditional model, goals are broken down into small steps and are often set by the rehabilitation staff. The goals for clients with chronic pain are usually concrete and obtainable. Typical goals might be: obtaining a higher level of physical fitness, improved mobility, weight decrease, improved physical function, improved ergonomic skills, and increased active coping skills. All of these methods can be used in ACT, but the overarching goal and the central focus of therapy is helping the client reclaim the life they have lost. In ACT clients set their own goals in the form of activities in valued life dimensions, rather than having their goals defined by the therapist. The clients thereby identify the course of direction for therapy. The therapists in the rehabilitation team function as a resource persons available to clients as the journey to reclaim their lives begins.

Values and Willingness

After the values compass has been established, the "willingness" to go forward toward those directions will have new meaning. If the client is asked why they do not go in those valued directions, they will most likely recite a list of obstacles. In the case of the client with chronic pain and stress symptoms, it is typically those very symptoms that are listed as the obstacles. In principle, the client is saying that the reason they do not move forward in valued directions is that they are avoiding painful emotions or what they believe to be physically painful barriers.

These barriers should be examined carefully with the client. What types of barriers are they? For the client with chronic pain/stress these barriers are generally stereotyped around a few verbal constructions concerning pain. Usually pain, exhaustion, and stress, with some variations, are at the core of these barriers. Although these obstacles are described as physical problems, they are in fact often negative private events with an anticipated consequence which conflicts with the value. For example, I want to work BUT I have pain. There would be no reason for the client to go into a situation which he or she believes will cause pain or stress unless there were also a good reason to do so. For the ACT client the good reason lies in the value based action. Willingness to go forward is dignified by the presence of values, not by the persuasive or social power of the therapist.

The Therapist and Values

Working with clients with chronic pain and stress can be a challenge for the therapist, especially when working with values. Values can easily be confused with moral judgments. It is very important that the therapist does not impose his or her own values on those of the client's values. Rendering moral judgments about whether patients should be working or on sick leave, or how much the social welfare system should be used, are examples of the problems therapists can encounter in this situation. Morals are social conventions that dictate what people "should" be doing, while values are personal choices driven by individual priorities. Social conventions may or may not coincide with the client's valued directions, and it is important that ACT therapists keep this in mind. The client with a long history of disability leave is likely to be very sensitive to judgments made about her employment history. It is therefore important that you, as the therapist, focus on the client's values rather than your own.

Additionally, professional conflicts may arise since many rehabilitation centers are commissioned by insurance companies to get clients who have been on sick leave to go back to work. Most people consider gainful employment an important dimension of life, but therapist must allow their clients to choose whether or not to return to work based on their own personal values rather than social convention. If therapists use treatment to openly or implicitly coerce clients into going back to work, this would not only be unethical but also therapeutically counterproductive in the long run. The therapist must do what he or she is asking the client to do, which is treating valuing as a personal choice rather than as compliance to social convention. Clients will be sensitive to whether the choices they make "disappoint" the therapist. Therefore, as the therapist you must assume that clients are making the right choices for themselves, even when they are not your choices. In the long run, however, clients often choose to return to work because they value making a contribution through employment. However, if clients sense that they are being coerced into making particular decisions regarding work, this is likely to prolong the time it takes them to make the right life choice for them.

Summary

In ACT the therapist weaves together the client's values, dreams, barriers, pain, choices, actions and willingness to form a sense of purpose and meaning to get out of the stuck place and get on with life. Living a purposeful, vital and dignified life can only be done if one is willing to experience some pain and stress. Choosing to move in one's valued directions is a commitment made with full knowledge of life's inevitable difficulties.

Assignments

1) Do the values compass for yourself. How well do your actions reflect your stated values?

2) Discuss your own difficulties in doing this exercise.

3) How does this exercise change your way of thinking about the problems you are experiencing?

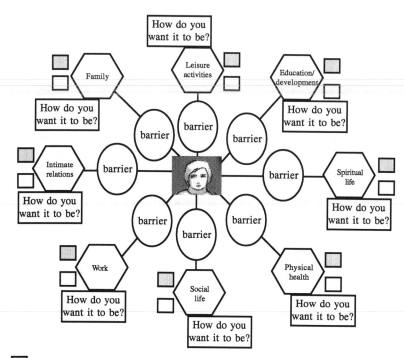

How satisfied are you with your own efforts (1-10)
Rank importance (1-10)

What do these hinder? Have in common? In what ways have you tried to solve the hinderances? What was the result in the short and long term?

Chapter 5

The Therapeutic Relationship in ACT

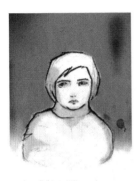

"I am very disappointed with people like you who have promised to help me but who have only made things worse for me. Nurses, physicians, physiotherapists, psychologists and social workers have told me what is wrong with me and told me what to do to get better. I did everything I was told but just got worse. When I told these different professionals that I was no better and in fact worse off because of their treatment, I could see that they were disappointed in me. I could have lied to them and told them I was better just to make them feel good, but I wanted to be honest. I wanted to get better. But instead of understanding me, they acted like I wasn't really sick at all. I felt I had to complain even more for them to really believe me. And the more I complained the more frustrated they looked. Some of them even avoided me and I could see that they were not listening to me. I would get so upset. I had sacrificed so much of my life treat my pain the way they recommended and things only got worse. Now that I have lost so much and am in greater pain than ever, the doctor has the nerve to say that nothing is wrong with me. After all of these disappointments with health care professionals, how can I ever trust anyone again?"

Establishing the Therapeutic Relationship

When we speak of the therapeutic relationship there is a tendency to think of the client's connection with the therapist; their trust; their sense of a working alliance. Psychotherapy outcome researchers often take measures of the quality of the therapeutic alliance, but the analysis typically focuses on the client. This is an inherently limited perspective. There are two actors in the patient client dyad, and the perspectives of both must considered when assessing the therapeutic relationship. Fortunately, as an empirical matter ACT is known to be relevant to both sides of the relationship (Hayes, Bissett, Roget, Padilla, Kohlenberg, Fisher et al., in press). Wilson & Luciano (2002) contains a specific chapter dedicated to this.

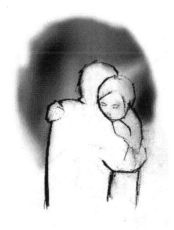

Many health care professionals report frustration and "burn-out" when working with clients who are stuck in chronic pain and stress. As health professionals we would like to be able to use our training to find out what is wrong and to help the person get well and move on with their lives. However, there are some clients who seem to be permanently stuck, buried under a multitude of symptoms related to pain and stress. This can be frustrating for both therapist and client. Therapist frustration can manifests itself in various ways, and if left unresolved can damage the therapeutic alliance.

Stuck clients are relegated to abstract, "official" diagnoses and treated as categories rather than whole human beings. This functions as an emotional avoidance strategy for the therapist, but the cost is the connection with the client. Progress becomes unlikely. In other instances judgmental threats of loss of income or employment is used to "motivate" the client to move forward. In the short run the client may more readily follow the therapist's rules, but pliance only adds to the sense of alienation felt by clients (who often tend to be high in pliance in any case). Counterpliance soon raises its head in the form of resentment and passive resistance, and the client's "stuckness" and suffering is only prolonged.

A good therapeutic alliance is a necessary starting point for effective therapy. This is especially true in ACT, which is an intensely interpersonal therapy. In our paradigm the alliance is the foundation that allows the therapist to rally around the goals of therapy the client chooses. The therapeutic stance is one of compassion for the stuck client. However, in order create to this alliance the therapist must be willing to expose him- or herself to the pain of seeing the suffering of another human being without necessarily knowing how to help. Your willingness as a therapist, to be present in your own pain in contacting the client's pain will help determine the nature and strength of your therapeutic relationship.

ACT involves two core components of interpersonal intimacy: emotional vulnerability and personal values. If you think about your most intimate relationships, you will probably find that these things lie at the center of them. The people with whom we are most intimate understand both our fears (vulnerabilities) and our aspirations (what we value). Similarly, in ACT we ask clients to share both what they hope for and the psychological barriers that are seemingly preventing them from realizing those hopes.

People with chronic pain are typically afraid of experiencing pain or anything associated with it, and they are also often afraid of examining the idealized, pain-free life they would live under different circumstances for fear that the contrast will only increase their suffering. The chronic pain client on long-term sick leave is both afraid of going back to work, and simultaneously hopes to return to gainful employment, as this is a component of their idealized life scenario. This classic approach-avoidance conflict usually keeps the client "stuck" in his or her pain symptoms, unable to move forward and unwilling fully to relinquish the hope of a return to normal life. Your client may rely on you for aid and support, and yet fear the power that you, as a therapist, wield over their lives and livelihood.

There is a message in these dialectical processes. We began in the last chapter with values, not with the client's barriers, but in fact the two are inextricably linked. In values you will find the barriers and in the barriers you will find the values. Thus it is important to keep these hopes, and their concomitant fears, in mind as you and your client work to build your therapeutic alliance.

The long-term chronic pain client is a special case in many ways, and must be treated mindfully if the therapeutic alliance is to flourish. For example, the client on disability has often already experienced disempowerment by being forced into treatment by health care authorities and/or insurance companies as part of the terms of their disability. In many rehabilitation centers, your job, in part, will be to determine if your client is in fact fit to work despite his or her diagnosis. It can be difficult to render this judgment while fostering a therapeutic alliance, as client and therapist can be seen as working at cross purposes here. The client is motivated to protect the disability payments for as long as returning to work seems impossible because of their pain. At the same time, the therapist must strive to render a fair judgment on the client's fitness to work in order to satisfy the insurance company which is, in this instance, the employer. ACT addresses this potential conflict by making the client's return to work an organic part of their reclamation of normal life, which is the aim of therapy.

The following dialogue with Bill illustrates an example of clinical positioning used in this model.

> Therapist: (Sitting face to face and very close) Bill, there are only two things that are important right here and right now in therapy: what is it you want, I mean really want, and what are you afraid of?
>
> Bill: What do I want? I want to get rid of this pain.
>
> Therapist: Why do you want to get rid of the pain? For what reason? What good would it do?
>
> Bill: Isn't that obvious? I can't live like this. All I have left in my life is this stupid pain.
>
> Therapist: That is exactly what I want to know about, Bill. About the life you want, the life you have lost and that you want back.
>
> Bill: I don't want to talk about that, it hurts too much since I know I can't have it.
>
> Therapist: Bill, I can see in your eyes that this is painful. You came to me for a reason; you want something more out of life or you would not have come here.
>
> Bill: Yes. I want to do more than just take care of this terrible pain in my back.
>
> Therapist: I want to hear more about what you want Bill. Tell me what it is about your life before the pain that you miss.
>
> Bill: OK (tears in his eyes). I miss my job. I miss my colleagues. I'm bored being at home all the time. Life feels meaningless. I miss playing

basketball with my sons. I miss making love with my wife and closeness to her. I miss going out for a beer with my friends.

Therapist: That's what I need to hear Bill. I can see and hear that these are really important parts of your life that have disappeared. These are parts of life that all of us value. They are what give meaning to our lives. That's true for all of us Bill, you and me, and all other human beings. Without those things, life would feel meaningless to anyone.

Bill: (Crying) I really try not to think of it. I try to think positive. But now, saying it out loud, I can feel how much it hurts.

Therapist: I can feel the pain of what you are saying, Bill. I can see and feel that pain, because I value the same things as you do, Bill, like having a job and working together with friends toward a common goal; intimacy with my partner; having fun with my kids; sharing life experiences with friends. All those things are what make us human being tick. They give our lives meaning and purpose.

Bill: This is really hard. You are reminding me of everything I was trying to shut out because I know I can never have it.

Therapist: What makes you think you can never have these things again Bill? What are you afraid of?

Bill: I'm afraid that I will just continue on this same path, suffering more and more losses because of this pain.

Therapist: I want to ask you something very important Bill. What are you afraid would happen if you try to move to reclaim some of your losses? If you tried, for example, going back to work, or rebuilding closeness with your family?

Bill: (crying) What I am really afraid of? I am mostly terrified to find out they don't need me anymore.

Comments on the Dialogue:

In this conversation, the therapist is looking for two things: what the client wants and what he is afraid of. The client seeks help by presenting the symptom (pain) a story or explanation (work, stress) about why they have the symptom and a solution (getting rid of the pain). Instead of engaging in the content of what the client is saying, we do a functional analysis of the story they present. The client seeks help because he wants something. If he had truly given up, he would not have sought help. The presentation of symptoms is the ticket to getting help in the health care system. By focusing on the function of healthcare seeking behavior we look at what the client wants. "Getting rid of the pain" is typically part of a larger context. What is the potential function of managing the chronic pain? Why is the client fighting pain? Embedded in the fight with pain are the client's individual values, which need to be identified if therapy is to progress. Since they are often values that we as therapists share, it is relatively easy for us to feel compassion for the loss of these valued life dimensions. By extension it should be easy for us, together with the client, to rally around the goal of moving in their valued directions. It is much for easier us to feel the compassion necessary to form a therapeutic alliance when we connect with clients on the level of shared human values, rather than focusing on symptom reduction.

The therapist has a responsibility to create the context of treatment at its outset. One feature of that context is to set the emotional tone of the treatment. Many therapists have been trained in traditions that insist on therapist opacity and distance. The reasoning behind this varies from approach to approach. In the behavior therapy movement sometimes such distance is promoted as a way to maintain a perspective of scientific objectivity. Presumably this objectivity allows the therapist to understand the client's problems in a way that leads to more effective interventions. This kind of training is typically not itself data based – in fact there are few systematic references to it in the behavior therapy literature. Instead it has grown up in some areas as an informal tradition through modeling and supervision.

Empirically, the facts are different. When factors are examined that predict good therapeutic outcomes, the strength of the therapeutic bond emerges as a key element of successful therapy (Horvath & Luborsky, 1993). Nothing is more important than establishing a powerful and meaningful relationship to the ultimate success of treatment, and it is the therapists responsibility to set the tone for that relationship. This should start from the first moment. At the beginning of treatment, the therapist has an opportunity, together with the client, to set the agenda for the course of therapy. What treatment will be about is described by the therapist, both in words and in action. Embedded in all of these introductory strategies are a number of ACT relevant issues. How the relationship is addressed is an expression of the therapist's values and the role values play in the therapist's life. Therapists can, for example, demonstrate that they value productive work. This may well mirror the client's own goals but even if it does not in specific terms it provides a model. The therapist also shows the role of acceptance, defusion, and a focus on the present moment in how the relationship is handled. If the therapist is asking the client to learn to watch their difficult thoughts without entanglement, it will be undermined if the therapist simultaneously models how he or she wants to be right about everything in session. If the therapist is asking the client to learn to open up to their own feelings, it will be undermined if the therapist conveys a subtle message that he or she does not want to be frightened or saddened by the client's own pain.

Power, Competence, and the Therapeutic Alliance

Our culture has dominantly embraced a medical model in the treatment of psychological problems. Within this model, the client comes to treatment assuming that they as the patient are "broken" in some important way and that the therapist is whole and competent. In the case of the client with chronic pain the person comes with a diagnosis of pain assuming some kind of pathology as the "brokenness." A power differential therefore automatically exists whether we like it or not. This power difference can play out in ways that slow the progress of treatment. For example, the client can play the one-down role in ways that are clinically counterproductive. The client with chronic pain may in some ways be motivated to stay sick, order to maintain payments disability payments and bonus health services, like physical therapy, that come with their sick leave package.

Assuming the "sick role" may also excuse the client from taking responsibility for pursuing therapeutic goals such as working or providing for their families. When a client falls short of their stated goals therapists usually take this as a cue to step in and salvage the situation in order to keep treatment on track. However, in adopting the role of the competent provider we run the risk of further reinforcing client incompetence.

Sometimes the larger and more competent the therapist appears, the smaller and less competent the client becomes. If improvements are not forthcoming the client may believe that they are even more hopeless than they thought when they entered treatment. "I can't even be fixed by the big, strong therapist" they, think "so maybe I am beyond help." Clients may adopt the story that they are different, and that individuals of their type are beyond help. Then, in keeping with this story, when therapy becomes difficult the client may choose to feel victimized by the therapist. Such role playing on the part of therapists and clients is counterproductive for obvious reasons; ACT therapy therefore to seeks to subvert the whole/ broken, sick/ well/ competent, incompetent dichotomies that underlie traditional models of psychopathology.

From an ACT perspective, much of what humans suffer from exists on a continuum, and every verbally competent human being shares the underlying pathological process. The psychologically healthiest person on the planet suffers from some of the same "stuckness" chronic pain client suffers from. ACT therapists often use to metaphors to help level the playing field between therapist and client, and to help clients see the similarities between themselves and the therapist rather than focusing on the power differential. An example of this is the "two mountain climbers" metaphor which is particularly useful when clients feel that only a person "in their shoes" could possibly understand them or help them.

> Therapist: It is as if we are two mountain climbers. We are each on our own mountain across a valley from one another. I may be able to see a path up your mountain, not because I have climbed your mountain, not because I am at the top shouting down to you, but because I am standing in a place where I can see things that you can't see because you are actually on the mountain. This is your therapy, but if it were mine, well ... I have my own mountain to climb, and you might be able to say something helpful about the path I am taking up the mountain. My advantage here is not that I am bigger, better, or stronger. It is simply an advantage of perspective. On the other hand, there are things about your mountain that I cannot see, that I will have to rely on you to tell me about. For example, whether the mountain you are trying to climb is the "right" mountain or not is a matter

of personal values. Only you can tell me that. And although I may be able to coach you along some path that I see, I cannot climb for you. So you see, you really have the more difficult job.

The Physical and Psychological Posture in ACT

There are many schools of thought on the quality of interaction in psychotherapy. In classical psychoanalysis the client did not even look at the therapist directly. Some behavior therapies takes on a didactic quality complete with a written agenda. In contrast, ACT tends to rely heavily on the relationship as the foundation for therapeutic work, and the kind of relationship that ACT seeks to establish is intense, meaningful, engaged, and purposeful.

At the beginning of treatment, the client knows something without which you cannot treat them effectively. They know their own experience. First, they know how they have suffered. They know how hard and how long they have tried. And second, they have some sense of a direction they want to take in their lives, and what they value. Without this information, you will not know them and you will be unable to help them.

This relationship posture is literally reflected the use of posture and interpersonal space. During the early phase of treatment phase of treatment, the therapist generally faces the client, and is seated relatively close. This produces an immediate sense of intensity and interest. The therapist should lean forward at times, as if reaching for key information, and listen as if the client was just about to reveal the keys to successful treatment. They will. When the client leaves the therapy session, it should be entirely clear that their experience, their story, was the single most important thing in that therapy room.

When barriers occur in therapy, posture can be used in other ways. For example, at times it can be useful to sit right next to the client, putting therapist and client barriers out in front to be experienced and examined. This posture communicates, without saying so, that you are with your client even when difficult material comes up – and together you both can look at it without running away or having it come between you.

Physical space: communicating an active engagement style. ACT sessions can involve standing up, moving, engaging in physical metaphors, and so on. The goal is to avoid needless defensive "comfort" and instead to engage with what is real, and what is present. The ACT therapeutic relationship is characterized by engagement and activity.

Ask the client to help you understand their experience. One way to structure a powerful and intimate relationship is to ask the client to help in doing so. The first thing we usually tell clients is "I need you to help me to understand your experience. If I am to be useful to you, I need to have some sense of what it has been like to be in your skin. I can't experience your experience directly, so my understanding will be imperfect. However, I need for you to do your best to transmit the details of your struggle."

Therapist: Elisabeth, for me to be useful to you, I need to understand your experience. I can both see and feel that you are tired, tense and upset. I want you to tell me about what you want. I need to know what you have lost and I need to know what you are afraid of.

State your therapy values explicitly. When we say that the therapist should express their values explicitly, we don't mean their religious or political beliefs. We mean their values as they relate to the therapeutic context. There are several values implicit in ACT and we believe that it is worthwhile making them explicit. Therapies are always laden with values. Sometimes the empirical clinical traditions have tried to pretend a values-free position, but it is a simply not so. Even in taking the time and trouble to try to "remove" depression or anxiety, one is expressing the value that it is better to be without depression and anxiety than to be with them. ACT is a values-laden therapy. In ACT we try to be very explicit about the values that drive the treatment.

Assumptions Underlying ACT

ACT is a treatment that works from a very particular assumptive posture. Here are some of the core features of that posture:

1. ACT assumes that, at some level, people hope, aspire, dream, and wish for a life that is broader, richer, and more meaningful.

If you assume that all people have values, then we all aspire to growth. Values are a direction not a thing. They are a "destination in view" that is never fully reached. In that sense, what is ahead is always a broader, richer, and more meaningful life. In the case of clients with chronic pain who are on sick leave, we can assume that these people want to "reclaim" their lives. Exactly what this will look like is up to the client, but it will generally include working, playing, and being actively involved in family, social and community life

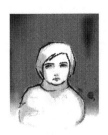

Therapist: Elisabeth, what do you most want?
Elisabeth: Of course if I could get rid of my pain, I would love to go back to work. But I know that can never happen. I have given up. I would also like to play sports again, but that will never happen. I realize that now. Sometimes, I even dream about traveling to far away places that I have only seen pictures of. But unless a miracle happens, I can never travel. I know I will spend the rest of my life nursing this pain.
Therapist: Elisabeth, I want to tell you what I am committed to. I commit my effort in helping you to reclaim your life's dreams. I'm not saying

that I know ahead of time how many of your goals you can achieve. I don't have a crystal ball. What I am saying is that, here and now, I commit to working for you and the reclamation of your dreams.

2. ACT assumes that under any and all conditions it is possible to live a life that is in accord with one's core values.

If values are directions, they do not depend on the situation. The form in which values are expressed may; the concrete goals may; the values do not. Consider a person who values being actively engaged in life. Physical exercise might be an expression of that value, but the situation can determine the forms this may take. Consider disability. As we move down the scale from being physically able to run to walking to rolling in a wheelchair to doing arm lifts while bed bound to talking without limb movement to blinking at an automated computer screen to communicate we are not changing the underlying value: we are changing the form in which that value is expressed.

To take a common example in chronic pain, a person can have stress and pain *and* live the kind of active, fulfilling life they want to live.

Elisabeth: How could I possibly do any of those things I have dreamed of when I'm in so much pain? You know my story by now. You know what happened to me before when I overdid things. It nearly killed me. I would never dare to try again.

Therapist: From what you have told me Elisabeth, you had already lost those dreams and activities before you got so exhausted.

Elisabeth: Yes, but if I couldn't even do all the things I had to do, how could I ever hope to do all the things I want to do?

Therapist: As I can see from the life compass you have drawn, you placed most of these things you want to do on hold, while you put all you energy in the musts.

Elisabeth: True. I have been waiting till I finished doing everything I have to do and thinking I would get to what I really wanted to do when I was done.

Therapist: And did you ever get there, Elisabeth; did you ever feel done?

Elisabeth: No, there is no end to the musts in my life.

Therapist: What if it were possible, Elisabeth, for you to live with this pain and work toward your dreams?

Elisabeth: That's impossible; I have to get my pain under control before I do anything else.

Therapist: But just imagine that it were possible, Elisabeth. What would you be willing to bear? How hard would you be willing to work if it meant that you could move forward?

ACT assumes that people have, in potentiality at least, what they need to deal with the psychological barriers to walking in a valued direction. Accepted emotions and memories are not barriers; defused thoughts are not barriers. Contact with the present moment and consciousness itself are available at any moment for a conscious human being. The assumption that humans have what they need to move in a valued direction is based on the idea that these other skills, while they need to be developed, as so elemental and primitive that it is more a matter of learning to let go of interfering behaviors and then developing them further than it is a matter of developing a set of behaviors that was at zero strength before intervention.

3. ACT assumes that some of the barriers to living a valued life are imposed by the social-verbal context, and occur most often in the form of experiential avoidance and cognitive fusion.

Typically, people with chronic pain/stress would be are responding to verbal rules like: "I can't go back to work until I get better," "Right now, the most important thing for me is to take care of my pain, or making sure that I avoid causing more pain." When the client fused with these rules, the behavioral repertoire narrows and psychological rigidity increases. Inside these rules is the message that it is bad to feel undesirable things and thus experiential avoidance is a natural result. These types of rules support useless avoidance behavior and needless loss of life quality. The person needs to learn to have these verbal rules occur without involvement and entanglement.

Elisabeth: How is it possible that I could move on with my life with this unbearable pain?

Therapist: When you find that your pain is unbearable, what does that usually mean for you? Let's take the example that you gave me from yesterday. You were planning on going out for a walk with Eddie so both of you could get some exercise. You have experience that walking and getting fresh air is good for both. You've told me that feel better your muscles relax and you sleep better when you exercise. The night before you and Eddie had planned to go out the next morning. But when you woke up, you felt a lot of pain and stiffness and didn't feel like going. You decided to listen to those feelings and that led to you canceling the walk.

Elisabeth: Yes, because I knew the walking would make it worse and I could hardly get out of bed.

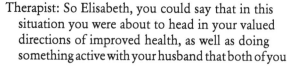

Therapist: So Elisabeth, you could say that in this situation you were about to head in your valued directions of improved health, as well as doing something active with your husband that both of you enjoyed. But then came the feeling of pain and the thought, "I can't do this, I have to think about my pain."

Elisabeth: Yes, that's exactly what happened, I know what happens if I don't put my pain first. I could loose control of it completely.

Therapist: So on the one hand, you had your experience telling you that walking helps build up your strength, helps your muscles relax, helps you sleep and brings you closer to Eddie; on the other hand you have your feelings that say, "I have pain, I am stiff, stay home, stay in bed, I could get worse.

Elisabeth: That's right I hear both of those voices, but they tell me opposite things.

Therapist: My question Elisabeth, is which of those two voices is your friend? I mean, if you look at your compass, and look at the direction that you want to go in? If you want to reclaim the good health you have enjoyed and reclaim doing things with Eddie and improving your relationship, which of those two voices will lead you in those directions?

Elisabeth: My experience is what would lead me where I want to go but the voice telling me to avoid the pain is so loud.

Therapist: It is important Elisabeth, to remind yourself of the compass you have made and the life directions you want to move in. When you have to make a decision and you get these conflicting voices, you should try to identify your own valued directions. If you really want to go there, your choices should be consistent with those directions whether or not the voices are encouraging you to go that way.

Elisabeth: Of course I want to go there!

4. ACT assumes that this social / verbal context can be altered in ways that can broaden a person's ability to choose a valued direction in their life.

Helping the person who is "stuck" in pain/stress symptoms involves altering the function of the verbal rules the person has made for himself or herself. If the rule "I love my work but I have pain and stress" is leading to absence of work, and if work is valued, the goal is to change the function of that rule. As this occurs new rules will be developed. ACT does alter the form of some rules in key areas. The rule "I love my work AND I have pain and stress" is more likely to co-occur with work, for example, and several language conventions like this are used to create more response flexibility. More importantly, however, ACT seeks to develop defusion skills so that "I have pain and stress" is no longer causally linked to not working even when this rule continues to occur.

The key aspects of the social / verbal context that are targeted in ACT are literality, reason-giving, experiential control, and evaluation. When these contexts are changed, verbal events produce less rigid behavior and the client begins to learn

- experientially not merely logically – that work and pain are not always incompatible, and that feeling of stress are not something to be very stressed about.

> Therapist: So Elisabeth, when you experience pain and say to yourself, "this is unbearable," what does that lead you to do?
>
> Elisabeth: I try not to do anything; I go back to bed until I feel better.
>
> Therapist: And when you have gone back to bed in the past where has that usually led you?
>
> Elisabeth: It's a relief first because I know I don't have to go out. But in the end I don't usually get better. I usually get stiffer. Plus I don't get out of the house.
>
> Therapist: So, when you let that "feeling of pain" and sentence "this pain is unbearable" steer, do you end up getting closer to or farther away from the directions you have identified here on your compass?
>
> Elisabeth: Farther away on most of those directions.
>
> Therapist: Are there other feelings and sentences like this one that have this same function? I mean, that lead you away from where you really want to go?
>
> Elisabeth: Let me think ... When I feel stressed because people are putting demands on me, I think "I can't handle this, I can't handle this feeling of stress, I'm stress sensitive."
>
> Therapist: Where do those feelings and thoughts lead you?
>
> Elisabeth: I back down, or protect myself and don't try.
>
> Therapist: If you look back at your compass again, does struggling with those feelings and thoughts lead you closer to or farther away from where you want to go?
>
> Elisabeth: Farther and farther away. I get more and more sensitive. That's why I've given up.
>
> Therapist: What about that sentence, Elisabeth "That's why I've given up." If you buy into that thought where does that one lead you?
>
> Elisabeth: It leads me to not trying at all.
>
> Therapist: Is that what you want?
>
> Elisabeth: No, I want my life back!

In this example, note how the thoughts and feelings that are functioning as barriers are never directly challenged. Rather their functions and costs are brought out and they are talked about in way that fundamentally alter how these events are treated in a social / verbal context. Implicitly, the therapist is modeling how to have thoughts as ongoing processes rather than treating them as what they say they are. That is the essence of cognitive defusion. Acceptance and defusion are present in ACT from the very beginning. A wide variety of specific techniques can be used to foster these processes, but even before any techniques are used they are part of the ACT therapeutic relationship.

5. The ACT therapist is committed to helping clients achieve the richest life (in terms of the client's own values) that is possible.

ACT is based on a fundamentally optimistic philosophy: not because optimism is a conclusion, but because it is a powerful and vitalizing assumption. It is important, however, for the assumption of the improvability of the human condition not be turned into another yardstick to fail against, on into the therapist browbeating the client about what is possible. There will be pressure on the therapist working with the person with chronic pain/stress to focus therapy on getting the person back to work. It will be very difficult to establish a therapeutic alliance if the client feels that you are going to coerce them back into the workplace before they are ready and regardless of their own choices and values. Getting "unstuck" will require a therapeutic alliance. Allying with the client around moving towards valued directions can set the stage for many types of change.

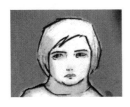

Therapist: If we look at work on your life compass, you have told me what you want from a job. You said you dream about being a teacher and want to make a difference in kids' lives – especially those kids that don't have so much educational support at home.

Elisabeth: That's right, but I know that can't happen so I don't even want to think about it, and I can't go back to my old job because it caused this pain in the first place. So I don't know what to do. I really feel pressure to go back to work from everyone. Is that why I have to see you? Are you going to try and get me to go back to work as well?

Therapist: What I want, Elisabeth, is for you to live as you want to live. I am committed to helping work in the service of that. I want to ask you again, as you look at your compass, have you been moving toward or away from your dream of being a teacher?

Elisabeth: I wish I had never told you that, because it's not going to happen. I can't even go back to my old job let alone a dream job. Are you kidding?

Therapist: No, I'm not kidding, Elisabeth. I want to tell you, that I am committed to working toward the directions that you feel are vital.

Elisabeth: (Crying) You are the first person I have spoken to in years that has wanted to know what I wanted from my life. Everyone else is telling me what to do, what is good for me, but I believe you do really care about what I want.

Therapist: What I care about doesn't really matter Elisabeth. The commitment I am making here to you is that I will work in the service of helping you reclaim your life.

Be Humble

We never tell clients that we are *sure* we can help them, particularly because that will inevitably be heard as a promise to remove their pain. There is relatively limited evidence in the pain literature that the experience of pain changes fundamentally for chronic pain patients, even if there is a significant increase in the individual's daily functioning level. Furthermore, ironically, if pain relief is functionally possible it is more likely when pain relief per se is abandoned as a goal.

The responsible therapist is aware of the limits of science as it applies to individual cases. There may be data on percentages helped, but typically clients come with their own unique convergence of difficulties. Bear in mind that there is no "average" client and more importantly, clients do not care about what happens to the average client, they care about their own prospects. Clinical trials cannot speak with authority regarding individual cases within the clinical trial, because the analyses are almost always conducted at the level of the group. They certainly cannot speak with authority to individuals outside the clinical trial, even probabilistically because we do not randomly sample from know populations either in the generation or application of clinical knowledge.

The commitment is to work in the service of the client. We tell clients explicitly that we intend to be useful to them and that we care about being useful to them. We tell them about the available data and its limits. ACT has accrued a reasonable database as a therapy and it is based upon behavioral principles that have been shown to be robust across a wide variety of behaviors and situations. The ultimate question for the client, though, is will this treatment improve my life? Only that client and that client's own experience can speak with authority to this issue. We make a commitment to the client to stop at regular periods in order to assess their sense of the progress of treatment. We tell them that they will be the ultimate judge of the success of treatment. This is especially appropriate since they were the judges of whether they need treatment in the first place.

Make a Therapeutic Contract

In the ACT model, the client's values direct the therapy. Making a therapeutic contract with the client is consistent within this approach. Clients with chronic pain/stress symptoms should not experience that therapy of any kind is being done *to* them. Many clients with chronic pain may feel coerced into treatment programs by insurance companies or employers, creating an even greater need for a declaration of intentions on both sides. This contract should be stated and reconfirmed as often as necessary. Often we find that it needs to be revisited virtually every session. The therapist should clearly state what the commitment to the client is and the client should state his or her treatment goals. The contract should clearly state what the working partnership is about. Within this model, the therapeutic contract can change over time. Changes will probably be minimal at first, and expand over time. Following is an example of how to make a contract with a chronic pain client:

"I have begun to get a sense of the pain you are experiencing. You have tried a lot of different things to manage it. From what you have told me, your pain has improved at times, only to return later. The other thing that I have gotten from what you have said is this sense of restriction in your life. It is as if your pain is squeezing the life out of you. What I am proposing is a course of treatment that is aimed at helping you to expand your life in ways that are consistent with what you care about. This will almost certainly mean that you will feel profoundly uncomfortable at times. Also, I cannot guarantee that we will be able to move ahead–but we might. What I do promise you is that I will stay with you as we move ahead in the treatment, and that we will only move into pain where it serves your values. We cannot do this properly unless you agree to the plan I've outlined. So I'm asking you are you willing to give this a try?"

Warn the Client that if Treatment is Successful, they May Feel Worse for a While.

If you went to the doctor with a broken arm which needed to be reset and she simply wrapped your arm up in a bandage and gave you comforting words and a pain killer, the appointment would have been fairly painless, but useless. Your pain might feel better temporarily because the doctor kept you comfortable but her treatment actually would have led to a life-long handicap.

ACT is a transformational approach because it is so fundamentally focused. ACT seeks a basic change in how thoughts, feelings, memories, bodily sensations, and the like play a role in human lives. Over the short-term this can be disorienting, and if chronic suppression and avoidance is halted, existing psychological challenges ill become more obvious. Short-term symptom alleviation that feeds harmful underlying functions provides temporary relief at the cost of more problems in the long run. ACT take almost the opposite approach by explicitly addressing the pain that is inherent in addressing human problems.

It is important to discuss with the clients that treatment may be painful as they move forward in valued directions. A question that needs to be asked often in therapy sessions is: if this feeling of pain constitutes the obstacle in between you and the life you want, are you willing to feel it for what it is and still move in that direction?

Assignment

1) Choose a client you are working with and consider how you would write or verbally express a therapeutic contract.

2) With respect to the therapeutic relationship, how is your therapy room set up? Can you sit close to the client? In what ways could you change your room so as to improve prerequisites for the therapeutic relationship?

3) Role-play doing the values life compass with your clients. Do you need to adapt the language of values for your population? What types of problems might you encounter when investigating values?

4) What are you own thoughts feelings about values that come up as you work with the values of clients? Are these thoughts an aid or a hindrance in establishing the therapeutic alliance necessary for working with your client? If a hindrance, would you be willing to have that thought without buying it and still work powerfully on client values?

Chapter 6

Values Assessment

The Cat only grinned when it saw Alice. It looked good natured, still, she thought it had VERY long claws and a great many teeth so she felt it ought to be treated with respect. "Cheshire Puss," she began, rather timidly, as she did not know if it would like the name; however it only grinned a little wider. "Come its pleased so far," thought Alice, and she went on. "Would you tell me please, which way I ought to go?"
"That depends a good deal on where you want to go," said the cat.
"I don't much care where — " said Alice
"Then it doesn't much matter which way you go," said the Cat.
" – so long as I get SOMEWHERE," Alice added as an explanation.
"Oh you're sure to do that," said the Cat, "if only you walk long enough."

Lewis Carroll
Alice in Wonderland

Beginning a Values-Focused Approach

In Chapter 4 we described our model of values and tried to show why it seems to make sense to emphasize it with this population. We also explained why we put it first. The issue of sequence is an empirical question and the final answer ultimately could setting dependent. There are effective ACT protocols for chronic pain that emphasize acceptance, mindfulness, and defusion early in the treatment process, putting values work later, but so far these have involved in-patient settings with programs of pre-established lengths (McCracken, Vowles, & Eccleston, in press). In that context, patients are generally "in for the whole ride." With a chronic pain population putting values first seems to be particularly important in contexts in which the length of time one has to work may be limited or in which drop out could be an issue. Early values work can be an ally in these contexts because especially when combined with a powerful therapeutic relationship it can motivate involvement and change and can help clients over the difficult parts of therapy. A clinical-experimental ACT values-clarification preparation with subclinical subjects showed this very clearly in just one session (see Luciano, Rodriguez, & Gutierrez, 2004).

If values work is being done early, however, as it is in the present approach, there must be a very systematic clinical approach to the issue, particularly because clients often initially do not know how to describe their values. If, as in the story, a therapeutic "depends a good deal on where you want to go" you have to know how to develop an answer to that question. It is not a common question. Thus, in the present chapter, we will revisit the issue of values in a practical and directly clinical way. The aim of this chapter is to present an orientation into how values assessment can be used to structure an ACT intervention with this population.

This chapter shows a variety of ways to use the Values Living Questionnaire (VLQ) to create a context for the individual from which the hard work of therapy can begin. Several variations will be described for both individual and organizational applications. The purpose underlying this effort is to identify and bring to the foreground the valued domains that make sense of why acceptance of pain is honorable and useful, not masochistic. The assumption in ACT is that each individual is a whole person with capacity to choose a valued life direction. Using the VLQ is a way of helping the individual to establish a life compass that provides a stable and long-term reference for treatment and the life changes that are occasioned by treatment. Using valued directions as a guiding light, day-to-day choices are more easily made that are consistent with the overall life directions the client is seeking.

Values Assessment: The Valued-Living Questionnaire

It may seem perplexing that the client comes to therapy with a problem or symptom like longstanding pain and stress and they are asked to describe valued life domains. Clients are almost always pleasantly surprised. We explain to clients that the perspective we work from seeks to understand people's difficulties in the context of a whole life. Sometimes problems become so overwhelming that it is easy to lose contact with the "big picture." We do want to know how the client has struggled, but seek an understanding of that struggle in the context of a whole person with other competing hopes, desires, and aspirations. Our experience has been that clients find this aspect of treatment useful and important (Dahl, Wilson, & Nilsson, in press), and a variety of other ACT protocols have been developed that take a similar approach (e.g., Hayes, Wilson, et al., in press).

One way to think about this work is that it is the verbal equivalent to the systematic reinforcer preference procedures that are commonly used in interventions with developmentally disabled children (Fox, Rotatori, Macklin, & Green, 1983). The technology to assess reinforcers for other populations is fairly weak, using such means as reinforcer surveys (e.g., Houlihan; Rodriguez, & Kloeckl, 1990). For verbal humans language produces reinforcer-like effects for events that are never fully achieved as a discrete consequence. In fact, if life is full of nothing but primary reinforcers, most humans find living relatively meaningless. The very term "meaningless" provides the clue to what is going on. Truly important reinforcers are part of a "meaningful" life – they fit with our deepest verbally constructed purposes. Having sex is reinforcing. Having sex with someone you are committed to is both meaningful and reinforcing, and it is *additionally* reinforcing because it is meaningful. It is about something (e.g., love, relationships, family, commitment, intimacy) and what it is about goes far beyond orgasms. Right now behavior therapy has no very good way to make the distinction. We think that values work is an advance in that area.

The Valued-Living Questionnaire was developed with the aim of establishing a context in which natural positive reinforcers could be found. As was mentioned in Chapter 4, the Valued-Living Questionnaire (modified from Hayes et al., 1999, p. 224; Wilson & Groom, 2002) taps into ten domains of living that are commonly identified as important, although there is nothing to prevent more specific domains from being added for specific clinical purposes. The instrument has shown good test-retest reliability (Wilson & Groom, 2002) and currently validity data is being collected. Regardless of the merit of this instrument in terms of its psychometric properties, however, it provides a systematic means to introduce the ACT values interventions, and so remains a sensible clinical tool.

Introducing the VLQ

In part one of the VLQ assessment process clients are asked to rate the importance of the ten domains on a 1-10 scale, including (1) family (other than parenting and intimate relations), (2) Marriage/couples/ intimate relations, (3) parenting, (4) friendship, (5) work, (6) education, (7) recreation, (8) spirituality, (9) citizenship, and (10) physical self-care. When discussing these values it is important to keep a high ceiling, because clients are often used to selling themselves short, in part of avoid the initial pain that can comes from seeing how far short their life is falling from what they want. It is important to tell the client that they need to think in general and constant terms rather than what might seem realistic. We make considerable effort in the instructions to remove conventional and social constraints on answering, by emphasizing that not everyone values all of these domains, and that some areas may be more important, or important in different ways at different times in an individual's life.

The following is an example of this phase of values assessment.

Therapist: Elisabeth, I want you to look at these values we have just written down on the board and give me a figure of how important each valued direction is for you.

Elisabeth: If I start with family and parenting, that would be a 10, but I would have to give my social life a 2 right now.

Therapist: Elisabeth I don't mean how things are right now or how realistic the rating should be. I just want you to tell me how important these directions have always been and probably will always be for you. We can look at your social life, for example. You have told me that having friends whom you could share life experiences with is something that is important to you. Is that a constant value? I mean, has that always been and will that always be important to you?

Elisabeth: Yes, but I just haven't had time.

Therapist: Elisabeth, I am not asking you why you haven't kept up with your friends, I'm just asking if your social life is important to you and how important it is.

Elisabeth: It has and will probably be very important. I would give it a 10, unless you want me to compare friends to my family. In that case I would give it a lower figure.

Therapist: No, I don't want you to compare any of these figures with each other. They can all be equally important.

Elisabeth: Then I would give all of them a 10.

In the second part of the assessment we ask clients to make an estimate, using the same 1-10 rating scale, of how consistently they have lived in accord with those values over the past week.

VLQ as a Life Compass

The original VLQ instrument consisted of a two-page instrument as described above. The VLQ in the form of a life compass was developed for clients with chronic pain and stress (see Figure 4.1 in Chapter 4). The ten domains, and two ratings of 1) importance and 2) consistency are the same in the life compass. The life compass was developed as an educational and clinical tool that can easily be used with individuals or groups. We have drawn the compass on a whiteboard for both individuals and groups, but it can also be done on a paper while sitting with the client.

Overview of Values Assessment Process using the Life Compass

1. Therapist and client go to a whiteboard or use paper
2. Therapist draws the client in the middle and 10 circles around the client that stand for specific domains.
3. Therapist and client identify and write in the label for each domain in each circle (e.g., family, parenting, intimacy, leisure time activities, education, work, spirituality, health, social network and citizenship – as well as other more specific domains that may be thought to be important in a given context such as "relationships with co-workers" or "relationship with the administration" and so on).
4. Therapist asks client to rate "importance" of each valued domain on a scale of one to ten.
5. Therapist asks client to write their "intentions" for each value – who do they want to be about in this domain
6. Therapist asks client to estimate how large a role they would like that value play in their day-to-day life.
7. Therapist asks client to rate how consistent their own activities (feet) were the past week with their written intentions.
8. Discrepancies between rated importance and client's activities are calculated.

This process should not take more than about 30 minutes, and may need to be redone several times during the course of therapy. We have found it useful to have the compass present in the therapy room and saved after each session. The compass can be used continuously as a reference with which all activities should be aligned. The following is a typical life compass result for a chronic pain client in the beginning of therapy, and illustrates some common problems faced by this population.

Reduced life quality: Feet are going in only a few directions. Of the 10 valued directions, only a few are "living" and "vital." The client has identified all 10 domains as important in theory but not in practice. Her feet are active in only a few dimensions. For women in public health service, it is common to see the caretaking dimensions (family, parenting and work) as vital and active, while the other 7 domains are inactive. In this case the hypothesis would be that the client has a "values illness" as described in Chapter 4. Our tentative hypothesis is that the "cause" of her being "stuck" in longstanding pain and stress is that she has shut down vital parts of life that are critical for health and well-being. The goal of therapy would be to help her to get her feet active in the other 7 dimensions.

I have too much to do already. Clients who already feel stressed and exhausted may balk at the thought of increasing activity in the other life dimensions. They may feel that they are overloaded with demands as it is, and would be more stressed by increased activity. This is a good time to discuss the issue of vital directions versus goals.

It is a popular belief that activities towards a goal can be measured in quantifiable steps. For example, if I have a goal of getting entering a marathon ski race, I will need to calculate how many miles of skiing I'll need to do between now and then to get myself in shape for that race. Quantifying steps in this way does work in many instances in life. This method of calculation helps us reach specific goals; however, specific goals are only a step in a greater scheme that is not quantifiable. A higher dimension of the ski race might be that the training required for the ski race increases life quality by getting the person out into nature, and helps the person become more aware of their body. It may supports health, and permit such benefits as better sleep and better ability to focus on tasks at hand. Similarly, ACT asks clients to focus on the higher, non-quantifiable dimension of their daily activities. In our experience, contact with these qualities is the exact opposite of "stress." It is this contact that provides meaning, purpose, and coherence in a human life. It is not a "demand" and nothing is being avoided: it is something being sought and appreciated.

How can we, as therapists, tell the difference between moving in valued directions with our pain clients and simply creating more stress for them? Again, we look to clients to be our guides in this vital phase of therapy. After identifying valued domains and expressing intentions in each domain, ask the client how they would know if they were going in the valued direction.

The answers vary, but most people can put this experienced quality into words with some work. The kinds of terms that come up are terms like "alive," "growing," "vital," "grounded," "connected," "present," "mindful," "being," "experiencing," "whole," "loving," or simply "living." It is important not to turn this quality into an emotion or evaluation despite attempts by our mental machinery to do so.

For that reason, any words that are applied to this experienced quality need to be held lightly. For that same reason sit is also important not to give clients a "right answer" or to overemphasize the purely verbal aspects of this task. Rather the goal is to have the client have a way of connecting with what it is like when one's feet and intentions are in alignment so that values work can provide useful guidance. Sometimes it is good simply to use a time when the client felt very connected with his or her values. For example, a father might remember what it was like to be there for his daughter when she needed him. Even if there are no words that seem to fit the totality of that experience, it can be used as a kind of shorthand for values work in other areas (e.g., "so, in this other domain, over the last week has it been more like the situation with your daughter or more like going through the motions?").

With practice therapists can learn to discriminate in the way in which the client talks about their activities. There is a certain emptiness that comes from a disconnection with values; and a certain heaviness or defensiveness that comes from turning values into yet another stick to hit oneself with.

Values Assessment Homework

It is often helpful to give the VLQ in the form of a homework assignment between sessions. It is sometimes said that ACT therapists avoid homework, but that is certainly not the case. Indeed, entire workbooks of ACT "homework" are now available (e.g., Heffner & Eifert, 2004). ACT is a behavior therapy, and there is very good evidence that homework can be clinically useful. What is generally avoided is formulaic homework assignments that treat clients as passive receptacles for information or knowledge. These are avoided because they can interfere with an open, honest, mutual, and interactive therapeutic relationship, and because they feed the idea that the therapists knows how to live the client's life better than they do. ACT homework is active, respectful, and exploratory. ACT therapists truly want to know what clients come up with and the homework products are treated with respect and receptivity. The therapist is always looking at the client's world in part through the client's eyes.

The following instructions can be used for the VLQ homework. It also is a good example of the kind of homework ACT emphasizes (this section is slightly modified from Hayes et al., 1999, p. 224-225. Because of the minor wording changes it is not placed in quotes).

The following are domains of life that are important to many people. Not everyone has the same values and this worksheet is not a test to see if you have the "correct" values, or to see how your values compare to someone else. This is about you. Describe your values as if no one would ever read this worksheet. As you work, think about each area in terms of both concrete goals you might have, and also in terms of more general life directions. So, for instance, you might value getting married as a concrete goal and being a loving spouse as a valued direction. The first example, getting married, is something that can be completed and obtained. The second example, being a loving spouse, does not have an end. If it is an end, it is always only an "end in view" – not an end that you can obtain like you can obtain an object. You can always be more loving, no matter how loving you already are.

Work through each of the life domains, even if they initially don't appear to apply to you. For example, even if you are not a parent, think of parenting roles you might choose to be in through volunteer work, with children in the neighborhood, and so on. Some of the domains overlap, but for purposes of this homework exercise treat them as separate. You may not have any valued goals in certain areas. You may skip those areas and we will discuss them when we next meet.

It is important that you write down what you would value if there were nothing in your way. This is not about what you think you could realistically get, or what you or others think you deserve. The issue is what you care about, what you would want to work toward if it were a free choice. While doing this worksheet, pretend that anything is possible.

We will work together to discuss these goals and values assessment in the next session. Clearly number each section, and keep them separate from one another.

The ten domains are: (1) family (other than parenting and intimate relations), (2) Marriage/couples/intimate relations, (3) parenting, (4) friendship, (5) work, (6) education, (7) recreation, (8) spirituality, (9) citizenship, and (10) physical self-care.

1. Family relations (other than parenting and intimate relations). In this section describe the type of brother/sister, son/daughter, you want to be. Describe the qualities you would want to have in those relation ships. Describe how you would treat these people under ideal circumstances.

2. Marriage/couples/intimate relations. In this section write down a description of the person you would like to be in an intimate relationship. Write down the type of relationship you would want to have. Try to focus on your role in that relationship.

3. Parenting. In this section describe the type of mother/father, or mother/ father figure you want to be. Describe the qualities you would want to have in those relationships. Describe how you would treat those you parent under ideal circumstances.

4. Friendships/social relations. In this section write down what it means to you to be a good friend. If you were able to be the best friend

possible, how would you behave toward your friends? Try to describe an ideal friendship in your eyes.

5. Employment. In this section describe what type of work you aspire to do. This can be very specific or very general. (Remember, this is in an ideal world). After writing about the type of work you would like to do, write about why it appeals to you. Next, discuss what kind of worker you would like to be with respect to your employer and coworkers. What would you want your work relations to be like?

6. Education/training. If you would like to pursue an education, formally or informally, or to pursue some specialized training, write about that. Write about why this sort of training or education appeals to you.

7. Recreation. Discuss the type of recreational life you would like to have including hobbies, sports, leisure activities, and so on.

8. Spirituality. We are not necessarily referring to organized religion in this section. What we mean by spirituality is whatever that means to you. This might be as simple as communing with nature, or as formal as participation in an organized religious group. Whatever spirituality means to you is fine. If this an important area of life write about what you would want it to be. As with all of the other areas, if this is not an important part of your values, skip to the next section.

9. Citizenship. For some people, participating in community affairs is an important part of life. For instance, some people feel that it is important to volunteer with the homeless or elderly; lobby governmental policymakers at the federal, state, or local level; participate as a member of a group committed to conserving wildlife; or participate in the service structure of a self-help group, such as Alcoholics Anonymous. If these sort of community oriented activities are important to you, write about what direction you would like to take in these areas. Write about what appeals to you about these kind of activities.

10. Physical well-being. In this section, describe your values related to maintaining your physical well-being. Write about health related issues such as sleep, diet, exercise, smoking, et cetera.

In-Session Values Work

In working through this raw material you will help the client apply the model we described in Chapter 4. You will help the client distinguish between choices and mere judgments. You will help the client distinguish between goals and values. You will try to root out efforts to please you or others, or to treat this as an exercise in being right or wrong. You will help client's over the tendency to treat this as an exercise designed to confirm their limitations, a process that emerges particularly when values are confused with preferences (e.g., "I want to be pain free" is not truly a value for chronic pain patients as can quickly be determined if you ask "and what would you tend want to be about if you were pain free.") Some of this work can be done in a worksheet form or through further homework exercises, but most of it is done in session.

In applying each of the distinctions above, careful questioning should be able to reveal the functional properties of initial values statements. For example it is extremely common for client's statements about valued ends to be instances of pliance – rule following supported by a history of arbitrary social consequences for the correspondence between rules and behavior. Said more simply, clients often are more interested in being a "good boy or girl" (or for some with a different history, the functional equivalent: a "bad boy or girl") than they are in being about sometime as a choice. Pliance, however, is responsive to certain variables such as social monitoring, and awareness of the rule. When the therapist attempt to detect and rework pliance-type responses the therapist would look for indications that values statement are controlled by:

1. the presence of the therapist, in conjunction with the client's assumptions about what would please the therapist. Relevant consequences would be signs of therapist approval and/or the absence of therapist disapproval.
2. the presence of the culture more generally. Relevant consequences would include the absence of cultural sanctions, broad social approval, or prestige.
3. the stated or assumed values of the client's parents. Relevant consequences are parental approval – either actually occurring or verbally constructed.

In these cases the therapist might ask additional questions such as "what if no body could know whether or not you had these values?" or "what if no one other than you could *ever* know whether or not you lived in accord with these values" or "what if your parents despised these values" and so on. When pliance is detected, typically the client can be redirected to what they themselves really would want "if it were a free choice," particularly by appealing to their own experience (e.g., "how does that feel when you say that? Do you feel more connected, more alive? [use the clients own words here ... see the section above]. Or do you feel heavy, afraid, self-righteous? [again use the clients own words.").

Examining VLQ Scores

After you have scored the valued domains for importance and consistency a number of different profiles are possible. Here are some of the more meaningful.

High Discrepancy between Rated Importance and Rated Consistency

This pattern is typically correlated with a lot of distress in the form of such things as negative self-evaluation, guilt, sadness and anxiety. It can be very difficult for our clients to even speak about what they want. The client has become so immobilized that even a thought of activity in these discrepant domains is painful. Generally what is happening is that the person is so high on cognitive fusion and experiential avoidance that the verbal formulation of an end-in-view simply feeds another round of verbal entanglement (e.g., with right/wrong; being able or not able), with intense psychological pain, and with avoidance as a major coping strategy.

Merely advocating activity is typically not helpful. Instead, we usually view this as a step in discovering the core of fusion and avoidance. This client is now ready for the acceptance, defusion, mindfulness, and exposure elements of ACT, which remove the blockage that has turned connection with what one really wants from a positive vision to a torture rack.

Extreme High Total Importance and/or Consistency Score

This pattern is surprisingly common early in therapy. Just as we commonly respond to others who ask us how we are doing with the response "I'm fine," so too clients are often more used to creating social acceptance than they are in creating real progress. If social acceptance is directing a client's life, it almost always begins to conflict with other values. Here again, what we have uncovered is the core of a fused and avoidant pattern. What does it mean to be disapproved of, and why is that being avoided? Often the effort to achieve social approval is based on a fused belief that one is unlovable, or unacceptable. The other processes in ACT will then help open the client up to the pain and narrowing of life that has come from fusion with this thought, form instances in the client's history in which they experienced disapproval, and from imagined future disapproval. We do so in order to help the client have a broader and more flexible repertoire with respect to thoughts about disapproval and actual disapproval and the feelings these both occasion.

It is worth mentioning that sometimes ratings of this kind come because clients answer these questions with little careful thought about the domain of interest. This does not necessarily involve deceit on the client's part but merely a habit of superficial positivity ("I'm fine"). In that case, a connection to social approval may not be strong and the rating may change with more scrutiny. The process of inquiring about the *particular* things valued within these domains often changes "fine" to something a bit less than fine. Problems can also be revealed by discussion of symptoms.

Of course, it could also be that the person really is living in accord with their values. In that case, treatment turns toward other targets or is simply not needed at all.

Extreme Low Total Importance Score

We have seen this profile in several client groups with whom we have worked. Among nurses treated for chronic pain, we have found very low importance scores that upon examination reflected adaptation to the perceived impossibility of obtaining anything worthwhile within the domain (Dahl, Wilson, & Nilsson, in press). For example, in the area of education, when asked about a low importance scores, clients might say that they are not smart enough to pursue anything educational. Note that "not smart enough" is unrelated to the client's experience of the importance of the domain. Whether it is possible is a different question and one that can be explored in therapy. Here we are just looking for importance. Some of these individuals valued this domain quite highly, but use "not caring" was a way to distance themselves from disturbing thoughts about past and possible future disappointments. We have also seen this among some college and high school students at-risk for academic failure. In this case going into the values in more detail will open things up, particularly as you assess for thoughts, memories, emotions and other aspects of experience that the client perceives as barriers to moving forward in a given domain.

Choosing Therapy Goals

Having collected the client's VLQ ratings, we examine them in detail. Whether across areas, or in a single area, we want to understand the client's stake in the valued domain. We want a deep sense of what it would mean to the client to make a difference in the selected domain. We also want to be sure that the client recognizes the therapist's personal commitment to understanding what the importance of that domain in the client's life, and to working with them to make a difference in that area of their life. We may not be able to completely achieve this latter goal, but we can make the aspiration clear to the client.

What we are seeking is a client value that can inspire both the therapist and the client to work together in creating a powerful and meaningful course of therapy. In essence, this then becomes the core of the therapeutic contract.

Consider Elisabeth, who presents for treatment for pain stress and the diagnosis of fibromyalgia. Using the VLQ we find a large discrepancy in rated importance and rated consistency in the domain of work. We find that one of the things factors that precipitated treatment is increased pressure for Elisabeth to return to work before she feels she is ready.

Because of the nature of the job training Elisabeth will have to sit for a couple of hours and not be able to get up and move around. Such situations at her job have in the past caused stress and pain. We elicit from Elisabeth other such events where she has experience these negative feelings and left work in the past and that she fears will happen in the future. We look for thoughts, memories, and emotions related to her role as a worker. If these topics are difficult, they become targets for acceptance, exposure, mindfulness, and defusion. These ACT methods create greater response flexibility, and as we see her flexibility increase we press forward behaviorally. When we are able to connect with the client around one of her central values, we prompt her to take concrete actions, using her skills to stay flexible and open.

Here is an interaction that would occur very early in therapy.

> Therapist: I can see how important it would be to you to participate fully in a job that was meaningful to you. I can see how much it would mean to the children you work with for you to really be there – not off in your head, checking your pain and monitoring your pain and stress levels – but really there, with them at that moment they learn to read and. What if our work here were about making that possible? Would you be willing to experience pain in order to help teach those children? I want you to know that if you agree to this work, I will devote myself to helping you realize that goal. Are you willing to have our therapy be about that?
>
> Elisabeth: Yes, but I don't see how that can happen unless the pain stops, or is at least under control.
>
> Therapist: Sure, and I am not asking you to take this on faith. Give me a period of time, and we will stop and evaluate how things are going. If you feel that the improvement in your quality of life outweigh the pain and stress you experience in the workplace, then we will have met our goal.

This intervention plants the seeds of the acceptance, exposure, defusion, and behavioral activation work that is to come. They link these steps to something that is powerful and meaningful. Therapy is now *about* something. A therapeutic contract exists.

Using the VLQ in Organizations

ACT applies as much to therapists as to clients. Indeed, the research literature on ACT is confirming that point (Hayes, Bissett, et al., in press). It also applies as much to organizations as it does to individuals. These properties open up ACT work to applications that are uncommon in the empirical clinical therapies.

The VLQ compass is useful for organizations who are stuck in a way that is similar to the way individual clients get stuck in their lives. Following is an example of how the VLQ can be used for a rehabilitation team working with chronic pain patients. The purpose here is the same as it is working with individuals, i.e. to create greater flexibility and a broader repertoire around problematic areas that have previously occasioned fusion and avoidance so that the group can move on in valued directions. Thus values assessment can be used both to help "diagnosis" organizational problems and to guide organizational interventions.

The setting is a consulting session between a psychologist and a rehabilitation team working primarily with patients with chronic pain and stress symptoms. The rehabilitation team consists of physical therapists, a social worker, a psychologist, occupational therapists, a nurse, and physicians. Here is an example of how such a team might utilize the VLQ.

> Psychologist: I'm going to put this rehab team at the center of this figure, and I'm going to surround the rehab team with life dimensions relevant to our task. I want to ask you to think of the rehab team as a single unit that shares values and that wants to achieve things. I want to know what the rehab team strives for and values. What is the meaning of your work here? Starting with the work dimension, I would like to write down the goals for this unit. What are the main reasons you come to work every day? What is it that makes your work here meaningful to you?

> Team: We want to help persons with chronic pain to live a better life. We want to help patients get off sick leave and get back to living lives they want to live. We want to see our clients realize their dreams.

> Psychologist: Is that right for the whole team? OK. Those shared values are the directions you as a team want to move toward in this work you're doing together. I am committed to helping you go in those directions. We'll get back to this in a while. Now let's look at your other dimensions.
>
> I want you to think about how important these other dimensions are to the rehab team. I'm thinking, for example, of how important is it for you to support team members who are parents. Is it important for the team to help its members be the kind of parents they want to be? Would that help you function more effectively as a unit? In a similar vein, how important is it for the team that team members take care of their health in the best possible way? How important is it that the team members have good leisure time experiences? How important is it for the team that the members continue to educate themselves and develop as professionals? Think about these dimensions and rate them on a scale of 1-10 to indicate how important they are to the team's ability to function in an optimal way.

(The team writes figures for each dimension on the white board, the P then averages the scores).

> Psychologist: Now I want you to rate your "intentions" for each dimension. How significant would you like each one to be in your day-to-day work life? And if it is significant, what might that look like? How might this value be manifest? In that aspect of it try to capture the core importance of each dimension.
>
> As an example you could think of how the workplace could support the individual team member in their leisure time activities. If you think that is important, ask yourself how such support might occur. For example, if a team member liked to kayak, you could look for ways to

feature that team member's favorite activities at the work place. The team might support him or her in doing that by taking his/her duties when there was a chance to do that activity. Kayaking might be brought in to the workplace as form of physical rehabilitation for your clients. In the same way, if family activities are important how could the rehab team support team members in their familial duties. Suppose they are helping a sick relative or taking care of small children. You might work together to create flexibility in the schedule so that members could be available immediately if problems arose. At the same time, these personal care-taking experiences could be useful to share with patients who might face similar situations in their own working lives. I want you to each write down intentions for all nine areas. Is it important? And if so, how would you like to see your rehab support each dimension and make use of it?

[The following represents the kind of brainstorming that they team engaged in as it worked through each dimension.]

Psychologist: Parenting: How could we as a team support our members' parenting duties? That is important.
Team: We would like to support all parents of young children so that they can enjoy both working and being parents at the same time.
Some of us could function as extended family members and help coworkers with their parenting duties. We could also help create a more flexible, family-friendly work schedule.
Psychologist: How could we make use of members' parenting experience in our work?
Team: Those with children could document strategies of how they handle juggling the competing roles of parent and employee. They could write about or present these strategies to us or to the patients and teach us by example. Children could be made welcome at the clinic.
Psychologist: How could we improve our social climate in the workplace?
Team: I guess we need to ask ourselves what kind of social community we really want at our workplace. How hard are we willing to work for it? Do can we foster a sense of community, so that we feel we're working towards common goals? How can we increase the level of trust and team cohesiveness while minimizing personal competition?
Psychologist: What are you willing to do to support these intentions?
Team: Well we could participate in some activity outside work hours on a regular basis, like bowling. We could support each other more when there are problems or when someone needs extra help.
We could take a trips together and get to know each other better.

Psychologist: Why would this each be important? How could good social network help this team function more effectively?

Team: The patients would benefit from a good psychosocial environment. We would work together better if we felt we were among friends We would tolerate difficulties better.

Psychologist: The next one is how could we integrate team members' spiritual lives into their work routine? What relevance do we think spirituality has in the workplace?

Team: I think this is crucial. Our workplace needs to have time a space to reflect over its directions and evaluate its content, just like individuals do. We need to examine and reflect over what we are doing. We need to position our work in a larger context in order to understand its value more fully. We need to appreciate what effect our work has on clients both in the short run and after they leave our care leave here.

We need to make space for reflection on the meaning of our work as a team.

Psychologist: So how could you work towards this intention?

Team: We could save an hour on Friday afternoons where we created a spiritual space for reflection on our roles as caregivers. We could do something non-verbal like go for a hike, or go swimming and just relax together. We could meditate together. A member could share a piece of writing that has significance for them in their work. We could process the events of the past week together.

Psychologist: How could spirituality and reflective thinking help the rehab team function better?

Team: By reflecting on what we do we could better see our mistakes and where there is room for improvement. By thinking about how we treat our patients we could better understand how they respond to us.

It would help foster a sense of community with each other.

Psychologist: How can we help members take better care of themselves physically? How is physical well-being relevant to our work as a team?

Team: We try and teach our patients the value of good health: of eating nutritious food, exercising and sleeping well. We should practice and lead by example.

Plus, if I'm not dealing with my health, I just feel much less connected to everything else.

Psychologist: What are you willing to do to promote good health in the workplace?

Team: We could encourage each other in our exercise programs and even do some exercising together and on work time.

We could create a nutrition course for the team where we learn more about, for example, vegetarian alternatives and heart-healthy cooking techniques. We already have a lot of knowledge here on our team. We

could help each other set personal goals, and encourage each other to
stick to our health regimens.

Psychologist: How would the workplace benefit from better health among
the team members?

Team: There would be less stress, tiredness and sick leave. It would improve
individual focus and productivity. We would be more credible as
therapists if we actually did what we teach our patients to do.

The psychologist goes through each of the nine dimensions in the same way,
encouraging the team to look at what is important and to look at what is possible
to foster areas that are important. Often these raise issues that have never been
discussed or even thought about. It is surprising, but people compartmentalize their
lives such that some very, very important domains are simply never thought about
as they apply to work. The effect is that work is disconnected from those other areas
and the connection to work wanes. Work becomes a burden, cut off from life. Much
of this seems to be a modern invention. In an agrarian culture, for example, work
and family are virtually one and the same activity. The family farms. Now specific
interventions are needed to connect family and work domains so that one involves
and enhances the other.

In the third part of this exercise the psychologist ask this of the team:
I want you all to think about yourself as a part of the rehab team and I want you rate
how much you yourself have contributed to making this workplace the way we all
want it to be. If you look at the domains that you have just rated as important in
creating this idealized workplace, I want you to evaluate how well that importance
was reflected by your activity in each area. If we call those activities your feet, I want
you to rate how consistent your feet have been with those intentions. You can all
come forward and mark a figure from one to ten in each area.

Following is a typical summary of the answers in each dimension (in this
exercise intimate relationships and family were combined).

Valued dimension	Importance (M)	Intention	Feet (M)
Work	9	Help people live better lives. Improved function	8.8
Social	9.2	Feeling of belonging Supportive, creative	2.1
Family	9.4	Supportive of others who are caretaking	1.8
Spiritual	9	Reflective evaluation of what we are doing	1.6

Parenting	10	Supportive of parents and welcoming to children	3
Education	9	Developing knowledge and skills in area of pain	8
Leisure	8	Support others and bring this into the workplace	1
Health	9.8	Support each other with exercise, healthy food and relaxation methods	2.3
Community	9.7	Workplace should be an active vital community	0

Results like this might be processed in the following way.

Psychologist: OK, we have here a summary of the values we share in our workplace. From the figures written here, we can see that we all share values that we deem important to creating a healthy, productive workplace. The intentions you all wrote in each dimension are similar in many ways. There were many different ideas of activities which could be promoted in the service of your shared values. In the third exercise, we looked at your feet with respect to your intentions, and we discovered that your intentions don't always correspond with the importance of a given domain. Our valued intentions at this workplace are similar and shared, but our feet are going in different directions. I would like to know why. Let's write down the barriers or reasons why we are not being as active as active as we could be in promoting our shared values. We can call them "stories."

Team: This workplace is unfair.
   We have no time for extra activities.
   We feel pressured to produce results.
   We're overworked.
   We need more education.
   We need a shorter working day.
   We need to have more clear instructions from the boss.
   We need better pay.
   We don't have enough confidence as team to be proactive in these ways.
   We need more resources.
   We need better equipment.

Psychologist: OK, these are "stories" are the obstacles that are preventing your team from pursuing its shared values in the workplace. Now I want to ask you about the strategies have you tried in confronting these obstacles, and what the results have been? Let's evaluate the efficacy of past strategies in each dimension both in the long and short-term.

[The following were the results of this process as the short and long term effects of strategies in a given dimension were considered.]

Social: We had a Christmas party last year and we went on a picnic last summer.

Results:

Short term: Both of those parties were fun and most of us had a good time, relaxing together. Short-term increase in team camaraderie and cohesiveness.

Long-term: In the long run, there was no improvement in the feeling of belonging or social support at our workplace. Seemed too disconnected from our day to day work.

Parenting: We invited everyone's families to that picnic last summer.

Results:
Short term: It was fun to meet everyone's families and children.

Long term. There was no significant improvement in meeting our goal of being supportive of workers' parenting activities. It was just one picnic.

Education: Representatives from each profession have attended continuing education courses this year.

Results:
Short term: the classes were very stimulating and interesting for the individuals who attended them.

Long term. All of us benefited members educational development. We have modified our program and improved it.

Health: We belonged to a national campaign last year where everyone got points if they exercised. We also have the right to go to the gym 30 minutes a week on working time.

Results:
Short term: We all made an effort for a week or two and that was good.

Long term. Only a couple of people go to the gym now, and those are the ones who would have done that anyway. No results in the long run.

Spiritual: Have not done anything

Leisure time activity: have not done anything.

Community: have not done anything.

Work: In order to reach the goal of helping persons with chronic pain to get "unstuck" and attain improved life quality, we have worked with the following strategies: a variety of physical therapy techniques like: orthopedic medicine, acupuncture, acupressure, body awareness training, Tai Chi, Qui gong, and different forms of massage. We have tried medical treatment such as injections, muscle relaxants, pain-killers and antidepressants. We have tried CBT techniques such as social skills training and cognitive restructuring. We have tried occupational therapy such as training in ergonomic work spaces. We have provided education the neurophysiology of pain mechanisms and the different pain treatments. We have communicated with our patients about their experiences with each of these methods of pain management.

Results:
Short term: About 50% of patients really are motivated to try all these treatments and they usually improve during their time in rehab. We can show that they improve their motor function and levels of physical fitness. About 50% feel forced to be here and many of these patients don't try at all.

Long term: There are no control groups. At the long follow-ups only a few per cent keep up with the exercises they learned here. Most of them return to old habits.

These were then processed in the following way.

Psychologist: If we look at these results, what conclusion would you make about the efforts and strategies used and the long term results?
Team: It doesn't look good. It looks like we are doing a lot of work but not progressing toward our stated goals. It is sad to see the things we have tried at this workplace while seeing so few results.

Psychologist: How does it feel to see this written down?

Team: It feels hopeless, like no matter how hard we work, we still won't get anywhere.

Psychologist: What if there were other ways to move forward?

Team: You mean besides solving all those problems first?

Psychologist: I mean, what if those solutions you wrote up here as ways to solve the "stories" we identified earlier are actually part of the problem? What if the team is stuck spending a lot of energy trying to reduce problems or to take away concerns, instead of using that energy to move forward day to day, moment to moment. Isn't it much like the patients you are working with who are stuck in trying to first get rid of their pain and then get on with their lives. What would happen if you just collected all those problems and took them with you on the journey toward meeting your shared goals? For example, we identified earlier barriers like "We need to have more clear instructions from the boss" or "We don't have enough confidence as team to be proactive in these ways." What if we made room for these ways of thinking, and still day to day moved forward in doing what we value? What's stopping you?

Team: What if we failed?

Psychologist: What are you afraid of? What would you fear about meeting regularly as a bowling team? Getting closer to each other? Spending time with each other in a meaningful way? Listening to the painful experiences of the overworked caretaker or the colleague in the middle of a divorce?

Team: I don't know if we can handle that. We aren't trained for that. We have enough problems with our patients.

Psychologist: What are you afraid of?

Team: I think we are afraid of seeing the human beings behind the roles we play, and of feeling their suffering. We're afraid that if we cared about them, it would hurt us to feel others suffer.

Psychologist: Would you be willing to feel that suffering and see that pain if it meant that you, as a team, could move closer to meeting your shared goals? And is it possible to do that even while having the though that, say, the boss should tell us how.

(Each member of the team indicates willingness)

Psychologist: Then, let's commit to moving toward creating this more ideal workplace together, even if that means putting up with some stress, discomfort, fear, or ambiguity along the way. Let's move toward our shared values and improving our effectiveness as a rehab team composed of all of these human beings with their own values, thought, and emotions.

(Each member of the team committed to this).

As this shows, the process of applying ACT organizationally is quite closely linked to the process of applying it individually. A number of additional writing are available to help clinicians interested in extending ACT in this way (e.g., Bond & Hayes, 2003; Bond, 2004).

Using Values as the Arena of Therapy

In this chapter several variations of the VLQ has been shown along with several applications. Identifying values with the individual or the organization serves several purposes. The main therapeutic use is that it provides a reference point for therapy. It also provides a source of motivation to make the changes necessary to meet valued goals.

Assignment

1) Do a VLQ on friends, colleagues or family members who are willing to do the exercise with you. Describe the results. What does the exercise teach you about functional analysis? What kinds of treatment goals does it generate?

Chapter 7

Identifying Components of an ACT Model through Functional Analysis

People act as they ought to act.
B.F. Skinner

Functional Analysis in an ACT Context

In an ACT model, psychological difficulties are thought to have to do with the interface between language processes and human behavior (Hayes, 2004). The general utility of language processes lead to a domination of verbal rules in the regulation of behavior as compared to other sources of control, even when this process is harmful – what is called cognitive fusion. This domination of verbal processes in turn leads to several other problems. The relational frames of coordination, time/causality, and comparison create the tendency to categorize, evaluate, predict, and attempt to avoid certain private events, which is called experiential avoidance. Experiential avoidance only increases the functional importance of these verbally categorized private experiences, and thus sensitivity to these events. Verbal entanglement leads to a loss of contact with the present moment, as the mind is drawn into a feared or fanaticized future. The self becomes an object of verbal categorization, as the person begins to see him or herself as a failure, or a victim, or hopeless. Meanwhile, there is a suspension of valued activities while the war within is fought.

All of these processes are evident in the pain patient. Clients actively fuse with thoughts about pain, such as the idea that pain must be reduced before valued directions can be pursued or the idea that their injuries are not fair; they avoid not just directly-experienced pain, but also the activities, thoughts, and emotions associated with it; they become drawn into a cognitive and behavioral focus on symptom alleviation to the exclusion of other behavioral strategies; they suspend valued activities in the service of pain reduction; and sink into feelings of hopelessness, depression, anxiety or anger regarding their inability to control pain.

The aim of this chapter is to link functional analysis within the context of the clients values explored in the previous chapter to these processes as they apply to longstanding pain and stress symptoms. We will walk through an example of functional analysis within the context of an ACT pain intervention. At the end of the chapter, functional analysis within ACT will be contrasted with a traditional CBT analysis of the same client.

A great deal has been written in the ACT literature about these processes and the techniques linked to them (e.g., see Hayes et al., 1999; Hayes & Strosahl, 2005). It is not our purpose in this volume to repeat that literature. Rather we want to show how to link that literature to the pain patient. In the chapter that follows we will then give examples of interventions that fit the components identified by the functional analysis as important.

We will revisit the case of Elisabeth to begin our examination of the role of functional analysis in ACT.

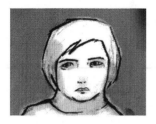

Therapist: Why did you come here Elisabeth?

Elisabeth: I don't really know. I just don't like my life anymore, it feels meaningless.

Therapist: What is it you want to have in your life that you don't have today?

Elisabeth: I feel like my pain takes up all my time. If I could just get rid of this terrible pain, maybe I could live again.

Therapist: Is that why you came here Elisabeth, to get rid of your pain?

Elisabeth: Yes, could you help me? If I could just make it more manageable so I could do a little more.

Therapist: If we got rid of your pain, what would you like to do more of that you don't do today?

Elisabeth: Right now, I would just like to be able to go to the store and carry home a bag of groceries by myself.

Therapist: Why do you want to be able to do that?

Elisabeth: I don't want to be dependent on people for everything.

Therapist: Why don't you want to be dependent?

Elisabeth: I've always been an active, independent person who helps other people. I don't want to have to get help just to shop.

Therapist: Is that what you miss Elisabeth? Being an active independent person who helps other people?

Elisabeth: Yes, I loved helping people: my family, my neighbors, and neighborhood kids. They used to come to me because I listened to them and could help them. I was good at helping people. They really appreciated me and life felt meaningful.

Therapist: So you miss that role you played, helping other people and feeling appreciated because you took the time to listen and help.

Elisabeth: Yes, I felt like I meant something then. Now, because of this pain, I'm too tired to do anything like that.

Therapist: I'm really interested in the life you want, Elisabeth. Not just going to the grocery store by yourself, but what you really want your life to mean.

The goal of ACT is to help clients contact their life as a conscious human being and consistently choose to act in alignment with their values, even in the presence of difficult private events such as pain, stress, fatigue, and the client's verbal fusion with their thoughts about these symptoms. ACT theory specifies a general kind of functional analysis. That is, the theory underlying ACT suggests what it is that we are likely to find in a given case. What justifies this idea, despite the fact that ACT is a behavior analytic approach, is that these processes are thought to flow from human language itself. In other words, there is a likely generic functional analysis specified in ACT, but within that generic model specific analyses need to be conducted to a) see if the generic model fits the case, and b) to provide important details about how these processes are manifest in a given case.

Functional Analysis: Assessment

Elisabeth brings into the therapy room three critical therapeutic variables: her presenting symptoms and their consequent losses in life quality, a story as to the cause of those symptoms, and a provisional solution, in the form of existing management strategies and ideas for new ones. These three items will be the focus of the functional analysis, but they occur in a broader context: the values underpinning the current "story." In Elisabeth's case, for example, the stated goal of "shopping without assistance" is merely a marker for a more fundamental goal: to reengage with the people around her. The desire to interact more meaningfully with her family and larger community has behavioral implications that go far beyond the simple navigation of everyday life tasks. In articulating her frustration at her inability to grocery shop, Elisabeth is revealing clues as to where her core values, and with them her motivations for behavioral change, really lie.

In the previous chapters we have put a great deal of emphasis on how to determine client values. Functional analysis in the context of values differs from functional analysis more generally for the following reason: many of the goals presented by clients that would lead to traditional forms of functional analysis are themselves revealed to be process goals, not outcome goals, when client values are examined. For example, pain clients want to cope more successfully with pain and the thoughts and feelings it occasions and this has led behavioral clinicians in the area to overemphasize successful pain coping in their traditional functional analyses. When client values are more fully explored, it becomes clear that "coping more successfully with pain" is in part a means to a larger end, but that means-end relationship is itself not being examined. Once the end is specified, a larger set of events come into the functional analysis. For example, instead of asking just what interferes with pain coping, one might begin to ask what leads pain and the thoughts and feelings it occasions to interfere with the accomplishment of valued ends. It is this very process that then leads to identification of the components of an ACT model in the functional analysis of the problems faced by chronic pain patients.

The following is an example of how a functional analysis could be structured for the client with chronic pain.

1. Identify the presenting symptoms and the personal losses and sacrifices in life quality that have resulted from attempts to manage pain symptoms.
2. Identify the client's "stories," or reasons why valued life directions are not pursued. Identify the client's verbal rules and other barriers to change.
3. Identify the strategies the client has been using to solve these problems and the events that seem to occasion use of these strategies.
4. Clarify the client's context for change based on identified valued directions.
5. Examine the short and long term results of the client's solutions, considered in the context of those values.
6. Construct a functional analysis of the client's strategies of symptom alleviation using ACT / RFT concepts (in particular cognitive fusion, experiential avoidance, the three senses of self, and contact with the present moment) and direct behavioral principles.
7. Begin to target the processes that emerge from that functional analysis
    Let's now look at these steps as they are applied to Elisabeth's case.

What is the Problem?

First we have to consider Elisabeth's presenting symptoms and their concomitant losses in life quality. Something is clearly wrong. Elisabeth states that she wants to move in valued life directions, but is repeatedly thrown off course despite her efforts to manage her symptoms. By listening carefully to the client's description of problems various keys will be found to explain why the client is stuck.

Symptoms: Elisabeth complains of frequent and unbearable pain, and feelings of exhaustion or "burn out" most of the time; she is tense and tired in all muscle groups, suffers depressive thoughts and an increased sensitivity to stress. She also has difficulty with concentration, recurring sleep problems.

Consequent losses in life quality: As a result of the above symptoms, Elisabeth says she is unable to work, engage in most physical activities, concentrate, or handle the stress and demands of everyday life. Significant life dimensions have been put on hold, and as a result life quality has deteriorated. Rather than attempting to surmount the barriers presented by pain, the client accepts a reduced quality of life.

Understanding how Elisabeth conceptualizes this life struggle is vital for the ultimate functional analysis in ACT. Clients seek help because they want something more from life, and cannot reach what they want because of barriers. These early description of problems are rich sources of clinical information. The clinician should listen closely to what to what the client says he or she wants: There are always underlying values present in this struggle. If the description of what the client wants is vague or general, like "a better life" or "less pain," work to reveal the underlying values on a higher level.

In Elisabeth's example, she initially tells the therapists that she would be happy if she could just shop and carry home a bag of groceries unaided. This is an example of an adaptation to reduced life quality. Underpinning that simple example, however, are important life values: the desire for independence, and the wish to help other people and to mean something in their lives. It is important for the therapist not to be satisfied with the presentation of goals at the initial, "lower" level of analysis, but to begin to discern and even to reveal the underlying values. Higher values will be needed as references, and should be used as a context for motivation in therapy. If the therapist did accept "carrying a bag of groceries" as a goal in therapy, for example, the adaptation to a reduced quality of life would be generally reinforced, and progress toward meaningful behavior change would be greatly undermined.

The other dominant aspect of the presentation of symptoms is that clues will be revealed about the type, amount, and focus of client problems from within ACT theory such as the domination of cognitive fusion, experiential avoidance, and defense of the conceptualized self.

What is the Story about those Problems?

In this portion of the analysis, the ACT therapist helps the client to describe their underlying analysis of the decrease in life quality. This is not done from an argumentative viewpoint, and it is not "one up." It is not being done to set up processes of cognitive disputation or reappraisal. Rather the attitude is one of intense, non-critical, but defused interest.

For example, here are some reasons Elisabeth provides for why she can no longer work or engage in meaningful social interactions.

Verbal Rules regarding pain symptoms:

I want to work but I have pain = having pain excludes working.
I would like to exercise but I have pain = having pain excludes exercise.
I would like to take responsibility but I am stress sensitive = stress
    sensitivity excludes responsibility.
I would like to sing in the choir but I just don't have the energy = lack of
    energy excludes singing in the choir.
I would like to meet my friends but I am just too tired = being tired excludes
    meeting friends.
I would like to get an education but I can't concentrate or sit for long periods
    = not being able to concentrate or sit for long periods excludes
    furthering my education.
I would like to meet my friends but I feel depressed = feeling depressed
    excludes meeting friends.

The purpose of exploring the client's own analysis is to detect the strength and kind of verbal rules that are currently guiding action. Once again this information is considered from an ACT point of view. The clinician is carefully noting not so much whether the rules are correct versus incorrect, or rational versus irrational, but the degree to which the clients is verbally "fused" with the rules they've generated;

whether these rules involve self-amplifying loops (e.g., as is common with rules related to experiential avoidance); whether there is explanatory flexibility or a rigid attempt to be right; whether behavior related to these rules is flexible or inflexible; and similar questions focused on the function of these rules.

How is the Problem Being Fixed and Going to be Fixed?

After identifying the verbal rules that form the foundation of the client's story, the ACT therapist should assess the strategies the client is using (and has used in the past) to manage his or her symptoms. Two questions are key: what are the strategies being pursued and what have the results been so far?

These need to be considered by examining the actual context in which coping has occurred, the nature of that coping, and the rules that underlie it. Generally, for the pain patient the key component of the "solution" distills down to attempts to eliminate, minimize, or otherwise avoid pain symptoms. These efforts needs to be examined carefully, and without a sense of criticism or judgment. In what circumstances have these strategies been employed? What different kinds of strategies have been used? What other strategies remain to be tried?

Typically clients are following the rule that successful avoidance of pain must take place *before* other changes can be implemented. This is clear in the solution rules Elisabeth applies to her pain problem.

(Pain excludes work) = First I must eliminate the pain, *then* I will work.

(Pain excludes exercise) = First I must eliminate the pain, and *then* I will exercise.

(Stress sensitivity excludes responsibility) = First I must eliminate stress sensitivity, and *then* I will take responsibility.

(Lack of energy excludes singing in choir) = First I must get back my energy, and *then* I will sing in choir.

(Tiredness excludes meeting friends) = First I must eliminate feelings of tiredness first, and *then* I will meet friends.

(Not being able to concentrate or sit for long periods excludes an education) = First I must be able to concentrate and sit for long periods, and *then* I will get an education.

(Feeling depressed excludes going out with friends) = First I must eliminate depression, and *then* I will meet friends.

These rules are unfortunate because the antecedents in these rules are not readily controlled, and attempts to control or avoid them tend only to increase their functional importance. Worse, the immediate effects of these attempts are often negatively reinforcing. A conventional behavioral analysis might be:

UCS demands   →UCR stress

SD demands   →R take time off   →SR- demands lessen

                                                       Stress reduced

This pattern of reinforcement impacts the entire behavioral chain, including the avoidance rules that supported it in the first place.

This is not the time to put an interpretation or behavioral analysis of these patterns in front of the client. Rather, it is important to "get the data" (both in the direct context – action area and the underlying rule area) so that a functional analysis can be made.

Assess the Underlying Values

We have already spent a lot of time on this section and thus will only mention it. The purpose of identifying client values at the start of the assessment is to establish a point of reference that will act as both a motivational force and a guide to selecting the most effective means of behavioral change. In ACT, the value of any action is its workability measured against the client's stated values (those s/he would have assuming "free" choice). At this stage, the therapist will introduce the VLQ (Values Living Questionnaire) and life compass to identify the client's most important vales, and assess the discrepancy between those values and the client's actual behavior.

Examine the Workability of the Client's Solutions.

In the case of Elisabeth, the therapist asks her to describe the strategies she believes will help her to regain movement in valued life directions. How will she move forward toward those intentions she described in her life compass? Because she is "stuck" in chronic pain and stress, Elisabeth will most likely answer that she must first get these symptoms under control before she can move forward. In response, the therapist asks her to describe the ways in which he or she has attempted to get the symptoms under control, and to examine the results of these strategies.

Therapist: Why are you here, Elisabeth?

Elisabeth: I have unbearable pain, I can't handle stress anymore. I can't do any of the things I need to do.

Therapist: What do you think is the cause of your problems?

Elisabeth: Along with the pain, I think I just had too many responsibilities, too much to do. I just couldn't handle it anymore.

Therapist: What do you think is the solution? How do you think I could help you?

Elisabeth: First I have to get rid of this pain. If you could help me manage my stress and pain, I could at least do the things I have to do. I also probably need to learn to say "no" and prioritize better.

Therapist: From what you have told me, you've spent a lot of time trying to do just that: minimize your pain and avoid stress. How has that been working for you?

Elisabeth: I guess not very well, or I wouldn't be here. It seems like the more I try to avoid things that will stress me out, the worse I feel. So now I can't do anything, and I still have pain and stress.

Therapist: Let's look at some of the strategies you've been using, and see
   if we can figure out why they haven't worked.

In an ACT-based functional assessment, you can categorize by problem, by
strategy, or by function (e.g., prevention, alleviation, avoidance, or distraction). The
question of short-term results is usually answered in respect to the degree to which
the immediate symptom is alleviated. Long-term results need to be judged with
respect to values, either generally or specifically, since they supply the long term
directions the client holds as important, but it is also worth noting whether the
immediate symptom goes back to where it was or even worsens. Clinical problems
tend to have a patterns of short term alleviation of the symptom and longer term loss
of contact with values and return of the symptom.

Consider a client who used the following strategies to get rid of pain. Each had
some immediate effect on getting rid of the pain, but when asked if he got closer
or farther away from his value (which involved doing meaningful work), the client
said in each case that he got farther away:

Solution	what have your tried	Results: short / long term (values)
Get rid of pain	Painkillers	helped at first / got further away
	Drank alcohol	helped some / got further away
Get rid of stress	Avoid demands	helped at first / got more stressed
	Tranquilizers	helped at first / got further away
Get more energy	Rest	helped at first / got more tired
	Avoided work	helped at first / got further away
Get rid of tiredness	Rest	helped at first / got more tired
	Avoided activities	helped at first / got more tired
Get back concentration	Rest	no help / farther away
	Avoid strain	no help / farther away
Be able to sit	Sit more at home	helps to sit / farther away
Get rid of depression	Antidepressants	helps some / farther away
	Think positively	no help / farther away

The process of examining these kinds of results is often revealing in itself,
without any overall conclusions being presented by the clinician in a directive way.
It is remarkable how long these kinds of struggles can go on without the client every
coming to face the overall pattern they imply. The client knows full well that the
specific attempts have not worked: what is missed is that it is the whole group of
strategies that is failing. Each failure leads to simply another attempt in another
form, but based on the same functional theme. By walking through the entire set,
the client begins to see the pattern and begins to consider its implications.

Generally early on in ACT the results of this analysis are not presented to the
client in the form of a conclusion that goes much beyond what the client him or

herself has said. We will describe this component of ACT later in this chapter and the next.

Components of an ACT Functional Analysis

The data collected can then be refined into functional response classes that are sensitive to an ACT formulation and to the client's contextual circumstances. This will allow the ACT clinician to link treatment components to the analysis, considering general behavioral themes and patterns, client history, current life context, and in-session behavior that might bear on the functional interpretation of specific targets in ACT terms.

From an ACT perspective these questions seem most important in formulating an ACT-focused functional analysis:

1. What is the overall level of experiential avoidance and what are the targets of that strategy (core unacceptable emotions, thoughts, and memories).

2. What are the dominant forms of avoidance and in what contexts to they occur, including
a. overt behavioral avoidance (e.g., avoiding jobs or school; sick leave)
b. internally based emotional control strategies, (i.e., negative distraction, negative self-instruction, excessive self-monitoring, dissociation)
c. external emotional control strategies (e.g., drinking, drug taking, smoking, eating, or self-injury)

People who are stuck in chronic pain and stress symptoms typically avoid situations, activities, movements, places, and persons that are either directly associated with pain and stress or that they verbally relate to pain and stress. The clinician needs to examine what the client does both externally and internally while attempting to manage, reduce, or eliminate pain and stress.

Overt behavioral forms of avoidance are usually readily detected, but the mythology of pain may make even clinicians who perceive the avoidant functions to fail to react to these issues. For example, sick leave is often encouraged by pain professionals, even though the data, reviewed earlier, provide little hope that it will be helpful. Some other forms of avoidance can be harder to detect. For example, emotional internal control strategies can include distraction from negative thoughts ("thinking positively"); reassurance ("do you think there is hope for me?"); negative self-instruction ("I am sick, therefore I don't have to behave responsibly"); excessive self-monitoring (constantly referring to pain scales to assess level of discomfort); dissociation (seeing pain as an external enemy rather than an internal condition). External emotional control strategies include some that are readily identified as avoidance (e.g., drinking) and others that serve the same function but are sometimes not recognized as such (e.g., self-injury). The forms can vary widely, and it is important to be sensitive to them so that they will be detected, and targeted. This includes detection in the clinical treatment situation itself, since a failure to detect avoidance in that context can easily lead to inadvertent reinforcement of avoidance by the clinician. For example, pain patients often both demand and get reassurance. Typically, demands are immediately reduced, reinforcing clinician reassurance. But if these requests serve an avoidance function, the clinician has now strengthened the very problematic pattern that is being treated.

Ignorance of avoidance functions can thus lead the clinician to participate in and to accidentally exacerbate self-amplifying patterns of avoidance. Probably one of the sadder examples of this is the use of analgesics. Drugs in the form of painkillers and tranquilizers, offered by the health care system with the purpose of relieving pain, can be a major problem for the client with chronic pain. These drugs are often prescribed "as needed" (meaning "as dependent on level of pain") thus drawing the pain patient into more focus on and control by perceived pain levels. The client often finds that the drugs offer less and less pain relief over time, but they continue to take them for lack of better alternatives. Addiction is a common result. Combining drugs with the alcohol is also common. With the daily structure and social control of the workday gone, drinking alcohol to gain relief from unpleasant feelings can go unnoticed.

Sick leave is another avoidance strategy that provides immediate short term relief from stress and that is commonly supported by professionals. It is easy to see how these "quick fix" strategies offered by the health care system can lead to a negative reinforcement trap. For the person who feels the pressure of stress and pain, a quick fix is attractive. For the professional, the immediate sense of having done something and the short term reduction in client demands serves much the same effect. The destructive long term consequences, like the gradual erosion of life quality or the gradually creation of an unmanageable health care system, are harder to see for both parties concerned.

3. Is the client fused with evaluative thoughts and conceptual categories, such as the domination of "right and wrong" even when it is harmful; high levels of reason-giving; the unusual importance of "understanding," and story telling? Is there a sense of resultant behavioral rigidity and the narrowing of behavioral repertoire?

Fusion with thoughts has consequences, but many of them are superficially positive for the client struggling with pain. Rules are held to rigidly because they provide understanding, and they provide some sense that what is happening is necessary or right, even if it is awful.

Here are some typical evaluative thoughts and conceptual categories for the client with chronic pain and stress. Note that the client's attachment to these evaluation often stems from the fact that if the evaluations are wrong, they are wrong. In other words, through fusion the client begins to have a built in investment in maintaining the current state of affairs, regardless of how destructive it has proven to be.

Evaluative thoughts	Who is made wrong if the client gets better?
I know my pain is caused by my work, I can't go back there.	The client.
The doctor says there is nothing wrong on my X-ray, but something must be off.	The client.
My neighbors don't believe I am really Sick enough to be home from work.	The client.
I have applied for permanent disability.	The client.
I'm a victim.	The client.
Nowadays, my only social contacts are the girls in the fibromyalgia club because we really understand each other. No one else really does.	The client.

Fusion with these types of evaluative thoughts are likely to be harmful, but they have a certain pay off: the client gets to be right. Unfortunately, for the client to be right, he or she has to stay sick. Being "right" may eventually come to dominate over getting better and getting back into life.

Therapists should examine these supports for fusion, such as the clients' evaluations about being right versus moving forward. Of course, any competent behavioral clinician would also look at the economic contingencies at play. Does the client need to stay sick in order to continue receiving monetary compensation? Are there other benefits in staying sick? Are treatments such as physical therapy, drug therapy perceived as positive contingent on the client's continues illness?

Note that detecting fusion and the supports for it do not lead in ACT to confrontation, dispute, and rational challenges. The client *thinks* he or she will be wrong, but the defusion techniques in ACT allow a very different solution. It is not literally the case that the client is "right" or "wrong." Letting go of attachment to a story leads minds to claim "you were wrong" but that very evaluation has impact only in the context of cognitive fusion. Thus, in ACT, we will not work to help the client *be* wrong, but through defusion to allow their minds to *say* they are wrong, in the service of life transformation.

Another major category of fusion is that of the conceptualized self. Inside the client's story is a version of who they are, such as "I'm a victim" or "I'm a failure." Even positive evaluations can be entangling, especially if they imply a definition of who the person *is*. In ACT these will be challenged indirectly, both through defusion and contact with a transcendent sense of self, and thus clinicians will need to be on the look out for any verbal formulations that imply self-identification with the concept.

4. What parts of life has the client dropped out of? Is their a loss of life direction, as displayed in the neglect of core values like marriage, family, self care, and spirituality?

The impact of avoidance and fusion on action is easily seen in the results from the VLQ. Typically, the person with chronic pain/stress will rate work, health, and education as important but will have put these dimensions on hold because of the pain. It is important to examine and clarify the nature and level of behavior avoidance in each life dimension, and the context in which is occurs, because these will help indicate the target and nature of appropriate interventions.

Besides the specific losses the client identifies, they client may also express a general lack of meaning or purpose in their lives. It is quite common for the person with chronic pain who has experienced great losses in life quality to appear "depressed" as a result. This depression is usually directly linked to the decreased activity in valued life arenas, and a result loss of contact with their own life. The less active a person in the various life dimensions, the fewer the chances they have to encounter positive reinforcement. The more the person becomes fused with the past and future, the less the vitality available in the present moment is available. The less positive reinforcement and vitality they experience, the greater the probability that helplessness and depression will occur. Reports of aimlessness or meaninglessness should lead to an assessment of the degree to which valued activities are being neglected, and contact with the present moment lost as the client becomes entangled in pain management strategies.

5. What are the specific consequences of having more direct contact with their experiences that the client is unwilling to risk? What are the core fears/private events avoided, and the feared consequences of defusing from literally held thoughts or rules?

If you have been considering the above dimensions you will have listed what the client is avoiding, with respect to activities, thoughts and feelings. The next step is to create functional categories for the content being avoided, and the consequences the client fears would result if they were to abandon their attachment to thoughts, rules, and avoidance behavior.

Let's turn again to Elisabeth to illustrate this.

Therapist: You wrote, Elisabeth, that you want to go back to your job. You said you miss your job, the kids there, and your old work friends.
Elisabeth: Yes, but I don't even want to think about that. I can't go back there, it would never work, I would get burned-out again.

Therapist: Just imagine that you could go back. Imagine that you are going back to work this afternoon, after we're done. What is it about that that feels scary?

Elisabeth: Why should I think about that? I know I can't go back.

Therapist: I don't know if you can or can't. But if it were possible to go back would it be worth trying this exercise?

Elisabeth: Yes, It would be worth trying.

Therapist: I want to see what it is in that situation that scares you. Let's just imagine that you are in a meeting with your boss and some of your work friends where it will be decided if you are going back to work.

Elisabeth: That sounds really scary.

Therapist: What frightens you in that situation?

Elisabeth: That they will say that they don't want me back.

Therapist: Let's look at that. You are in the meeting and your boss asks you, "Elisabeth, what do you want to do?" What is your answer?

Elisabeth: That I don't know.

Therapist: Where does saying "I don't know" get you?

Elisabeth: That I don't need to answer.

Therapist: What would be scary about saying out loud in that meeting that what you want is to come back to work?

Elisabeth: Because maybe they don't want me back.

Therapist: How are you going to know that if you don't tell them what you want to do?

Elisabeth: I think it would be better to have the union people there. They can speak for me. They know my rights.

Therapist: I am sure they do. But this situation is about you and what you want, and what is scary about telling your employer and your work friends that you want to come back.

Elisabeth: I told you: they might not want me.

Therapist: They may want you or they may not want you Elisabeth. But if you tell them what you want, you will give yourself a chance to get it. What you are doing is betting on the dead horse. You're not giving yourself the chance to win if you don't bet on the live horse.

Elisabeth: Why would they want me anyway? They have a substitute right now who is younger and healthier than I am.

Therapist: What are you really afraid of here?

Elisabeth: I am afraid of showing them what I really want. If I really told them how I feel, that I miss them every day and really want to come back, I'm afraid they would turn their backs on me. (Crying) I want so much have a job again and feel like a part of something. I'm afraid they won't let me have that.

Therapist: So, to avoid being rejected, you reject them first?

Elisabeth: Yes, it looks like that's what I'm doing.

Therapist: Are you doing that in the other categories as well Elisabeth? Is that what you are doing in your intimate relationship dimension, in the social network dimension?

Elisabeth: I guess so. Yeah, I'm afraid there too, that they don't want me any more. I have just given up. I don't give anyone a chance.

Therapist: So, in how many of these areas are you betting on the dead horse?

Elisabeth: All of them, I guess.

Clients with chronic pain and stress typically express negative expectations about pain becoming worse, or even unbearable. They have learned various strategies and rules that they believe exert some control over pain. They believe letting go of those control strategies might result in a catastrophe in the form of uncontrollable pain. Pain clients have already often experienced significant losses in life quality since pain entered their lives. In their experience the pain has usually only gotten worse, not better, and it now occupies most life dimensions. A common fear is that this process will continue to unfold inexorably.

Acceptance and defusion are not obvious alternatives when facing pain. Pain is by its nature aversive and serves as a call to action. Acute pain signals danger and functions to protect us. The same can be said for the stress reaction. A stress reaction is also an alarm system that calls for mobilization. The alarm system in itself is an unconditioned response. Problems arise as this alarm system becomes conditioned to a variety of situations where it is not called for, and worse, as responding to the alarm system leads to a more sensitive alarm system. This might be similar to an oversensitive car alarm. You want your car alarm to set off when someone is breaking into your car but you don't want it going off when you are sitting in a job interview.

Acceptance and defusion superficially appear to make negative outcomes more likely, even though we know as a scientific matter the exact opposite is true. Deliberate coping strategies drawn the client into more focus on and behavioral control by pain. Avoidance patterns result in serious mutilation of life quality. Nevertheless, logically it seems that letting go of this process of "control" will lead to pain being "out of control" and the experienced bad outcomes from inappropriate control strategies lead to yet another round of such strategies.

As initial assessment concludes in ACT, it often begins to fold naturally into a confrontation of the harmful control agenda. The following is an example.

Therapist: What do you believe would happen, Elisabeth, if you stopped trying to control your pain? I mean stopped taking the painkillers and stopped being on sick leave, and started doing all those things you want to do?

Elisabeth: If I did that, I'm afraid that my pain would get totally out of control. Who knows what would happen. Things are so bad now; I don't want everything to get worse.

Therapist: I don't want you to believe me, Elisabeth, but only look at your own experience about how these strategies have worked in getting you closer to getting your life back.

Elisabeth: I see that they have gotten me further away, but I am afraid of losing everything if I stopped trying to control my pain.

Therapist: Maybe it's like this. Imagine a situation where there was a monster and a person like you who were in a tug-of-war. The monster and the person were pulling frantically on each end of the rope, and in-between them was a ravine. Both the monster and the person were pulling like their life depended on it because neither wanted to fall into that ravine. Can you see yourself in this story? The monster is your pain and the person is you, pulling frantically so the monster doesn't pull you into that ravine.

Elisabeth: Yes, that's just what it feels like. I have to fight with my life to keep from falling into the pit. That fight is so hard it squeezes the life out of me.

Therapist: That is what I see you doing also, Elisabeth. You are fighting the pain so hard, just like with the monster, and that fight has already cost you much of your life.

Elisabeth: That's what I said; I have no choice but to fight that monster.

Therapist: Oh, but you do have a choice. You know what else you could do? Let go of the rope. Just let go and stop the fight.

Elisabeth: Just let go? That's it?

Therapist: That's it. Let go of the rope.

Elisabeth: What if the monster comes running after me? Overtakes me and all parts of my life?

Therapist: What if the pain you are experiencing is not the enemy, even if it looks and feels awful? What if it were the case that it is the fight against experiencing pain that is harmful and traumatic?

Elisabeth: You mean that it isn't my pain that is the monster but my fighting it that is the monster?

Therapist: Take a look at your life. When you were working and living an active life, you also had pain.

Elisabeth: Yes, that's how it all started, that's what caused my stress and pain.

Therapist: That may well be, but when you stopped doing all those things that you think caused your pain, and you started focusing on fighting your pain, did it get better or worse?

Elisabeth: It got worse.

Therapist: What conclusion do you draw from that? What happened when you made your pain the enemy and spent most of your time fighting it?

Elisabeth: It became more important than everything else. It influenced my
    whole life.
Therapist: Just like the monster?
Elisabeth: … Are you telling me I should make friends with the monster?
Therapist: I am not actually telling you to do anything Elisabeth. I would
        just ask that you look at your own experience.

We will pick up on this line of work in ACT in the next chapter.

Putting These Elements Together

The components of an ACT functional analysis of chronic pain are shown in
Figure 7.1. In the context of initial pain and stress, the client has fused with pain
related thoughts and used experiential avoidance strategies as a dominant form of
pain-related coping. These processes have been strengthened by such factors as
initial negative reinforcement but a reduction in pain or stress (due to avoidance)
and social / verbal support (e.g., support for being right; having a coherent
explanation). As these verbal regulatory processes have dominated, the person has
lost effective contact with the vitality the present moment affords, and they have
become more entangled with their story about themselves and their life. Meanwhile,
a valued life is put on hold, often so completely that the person is not really clear
about what they want in their lives. This entire package is resulting in more rigidity
and a loss of vitality, which further increase negative thoughts and feelings, leading
to still more avoidance and fusion, and still less values based action. A self-
amplifying loop emerges as the person slides into chronic pain syndrome.

This analysis shares some features with a traditional CBT functional analysis.
Situational antecedents and consequences are still relevant; thoughts and feelings
are still relevant; and so on. What is different is that the form of difficult content
is not a focus of the analysis. Thoughts are not parsed into rational or irrational
varieties. Pain or stress is not presumed to be something that must be diminished.
Instead, the key issue is one of function, and the analysis and the treatment
components tied to it are centered on creating more flexible forms of responding
linked to the larger life values of importance to the client.

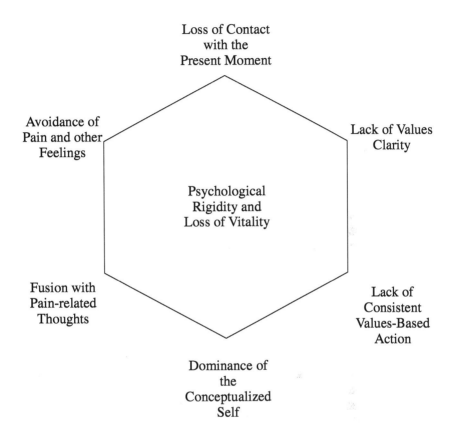

Figure 7.1. A model of an ACT formulation of chronic pain.

Chapter 8

ACT Interventions

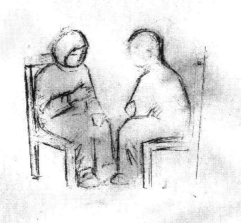

In this chapter we will give examples of how to link ACT interventions to the analysis presented in the last chapter, using the case of Elisabeth as our organizational outline. There are a very wide variety of ACT interventions methods (e.g., Hayes et al., 1999; Hayes & Strosahl, 2005; Wilson & Luciano, 2002), many of which are of obvious and direct relevance to pain. It is not our purpose to repeat those here, but rather to show how they are relevant to this clinical target.

Undermining Avoidance and Fusion

In the ACT model of chronic pain, avoidance and fusion are two pathological lynchpins for a life-narrowing struggle. Often as assessment itself proceeds, the ACT therapist will begin compassionately to reflect back to client what they themselves are saying about the unworkablility of their current strategies. The short-term functional analysis usually shows that the client does effectively alleviate pain and stress by using avoidance strategies. However, when we use the life compass as a reference point and we apply a larger metric of flexibility and vitality we see the long term outcome of avoiding pain and stress has been a reduction in overall life quality.

It is the client's experience of workability that determines the utility of avoidance and fusion, not the judgment of the therapist. But it is remarkable how short-term effects and language itself can deflect the client from facing what they themselves experience to be true.

Exploring the client's experience in this area has been called "creative hopelessness." The term is confusing if "hopelessness" is taken to be a feeling or thought. This process does not feel hopeless (if anything it usually feels oddly hopeful) and it is not about convincing clients that they are hopeless. It is something more akin to laying down a heavy burden that cannot, and need not, be carried. Carrying this burden is hopeless and useless – seeing that it not longer needs to be carried is freeing, hopeful, and liberating. "Creative hopelessness" is like that.

Therapist: Elisabeth, when you look at all you have done to get rid of your pain and feelings of stress and tiredness, where has it gotten you? You have far more experience than I do about what you have done and how it has served you.

Elisabeth: It is really hard to see my life laid out like that [in the life compass]. I knew this but it is painful to see so clearly on that board how much I have done and how hard I have tried. For what? I'm much worse off now than when I started.

Therapist: What is your conclusion about the types of strategies you have tried? We could look at them category by category. Some of these strategies, like being on sick leave and resting, were meant to protect you from pain and stress. Is that right?

Elisabeth: Yes, I stayed home from work and rested because I knew that I would get pain and stress if I went to work.

Therapist: So, you could say that you avoided physical and mental strain as a strategy to prevent pain and stress and that led to, as you wrote here, an immediate reduction of demands. But in the long run what happened?

Elisabeth: I got more stressed out and had more pain in the long run. It's funny, but it seems like I got used to the situation. Before this pain I could do hundreds a things a day, but today, when I do less, I have more stress.

Therapist: So, what is your conclusion about using strategies of avoidance to prevent pain and stress?

Elisabeth: That they only help for the moment and they make life harder in the end.

Therapist: What do you mean by harder?

Elisabeth: I mean that avoiding work and other activities makes it harder to go back. Everything feels like a chore and it's just easier not to do anything. But it makes me depressed.

Therapist: What about other strategies you used to symptom alleviation, like painkillers and muscle relaxants? How did they work for you with respect to getting closer to the life you want to live?

Elisabeth: At first they worked pretty well. When I was working I could take a pill if I started getting pain in my neck and shoulders, and I could keep going. But as soon as I started taking them regularly they stopped working. I took them anyway because I was afraid I'd have more pain if I stopped. But in the long run, taking more and more painkillers and muscle relaxants only made me more drowsy and tired. They have not helped me move forward in my life.

Therapist: What about the strategies you have used to help yourself with negative thoughts. You described that when you had depressive thoughts you tried to use strategies like positive thinking as a distraction.

Elisabeth: I have always tried to be a happy person and look on the bright side of things. I read in a magazine about stress management and mental training, and I try to practice positive thinking.

Therapist: How do you do that?

Elisabeth: Whenever I started to feel sad about not being at my job, I just started thinking about all the good things in my life. They said in the magazine to make a list of what I like about myself and put it on the refrigerator. So when I felt sad I would go there and read those things out loud. I tried to chase away the bad thoughts with good thoughts.

Therapist: How did that work for you?

Elisabeth: It was pretty pathetic! Can you picture me standing by the refrigerator ten times a day reading that list? Maybe it helped to distract me somewhat. But it sure didn't get me closer to what I wanted to be doing. Maybe I wasn't doing it right. Do you know a better way?

Therapist: No Elisabeth, in fact I have never heard of any way we human beings can get rid of negative thoughts. You also mentioned that you thought you needed to say "no" and make new priorities in your life. What did you mean by that?

Elisabeth: That is one of the reasons why I'm sitting here. I can never say no to anyone and I end up having to do all kinds of things I don't want to do because I can't say no. I just don't have very good self-confidence. If I just could assert myself better and get more self-confidence, maybe I could go on with my life. Could you help me with that?

Therapist: How have you tried to improve your self-confidence?

Elisabeth: I have tried to show people when I am mad and irritated at them. I say more what I think.

Therapist: And what has that led to? Have you gotten closer, for example, to the types of close relationships that you want?

Elisabeth: No, I've just made more conflicts and trouble. I thought that the problem was that I just said yes to everything, but there must be something else.

Therapist: OK, Elisabeth, let's try and summarize here. On the one hand, you have many years of experience trying to prevent or get rid of your pain and stress by avoiding things like work and physical or mental strain. Your experience tells you that avoidance and suppression using drugs or positive thinking only has a short-term effect, but in the long term you are worse off than before. Is that correct?

Elisabeth: Yeah, that's exactly my experience. How pathetic.

Therapist: On the other hand, despite this experience, your feelings tell you should try something else. When you came through that door, you wanted help getting rid of the pain and increasing self-confidence.

Elisabeth: Well, I try to stay an optimist. I can't just give up. Maybe someday, they will figure out the cause of my pain. I thought maybe you could help me.

Therapist: That is what I meant Elisabeth. On the one hand you have more experience that anyone else with your pain and what you have done to try and get rid of it. And no one knows better than you that trying to avoid pain has mostly led to undesirable outcomes. Yet at the same time, you have feelings and thoughts encouraging you keep trying new ways to avoid pain.

Elisabeth: Are you telling me to give up, that it is hopeless?

Therapist: I'm not telling you anything. But what does your experience tell you? How is that different from what your feelings tell you? Which of those two voices do you think will steer you closer to the life you want to be living?

Elisabeth: My experience tells me that I will never get rid of my pain if I keep doing what I've done in the past, but my feelings tell me to keep trying to find a cure, a new doctor, or new research that will take care of the pain once and for all. Does that mean I should try and just live with my pain? I don't know if I can do that.

Therapist: I am only trying to help you see from the perspective of where you want your life to be going, which of these strategies would help you get there. You are the one with the experience.

Elisabeth: I know now these strategies don't work but I don't know what else to do.

Different metaphors can be helpful to the client to provide a common sense model for more complex processes. The paradoxical effects of avoidance and fusion occur precisely because what is logical is not necessarily functional. Metaphors can cut through the verbal complexity and help the client see what has been happening, and what, by implication, they may need to do differently. The "Baby Tiger" is an example:

Imagine that when you go home tonight that you found a baby tiger in your kitchen, the little tiger is a cute little animal but he also snarls at you like he wants something. You look in the refrigerator and find some meat to give him. He is satisfied a short while but then comes back again, and again and again, wanting more and more each time. Soon when you look you have nothing more to give him and when you turn around to look at him he has become, HUGE, and there is only you left to eat. Imagine that the little tiger was your pain from the beginning and that you sacrificed one activity after the other in your life to soothe the tiger, or keep the pain quiet. The pain only quiets down temporarily and gets larger and more intensive over time occupying a greater and greater place in my life. In the end the pain overshadows all other parts of life and you spend all your time trying to control it. Does that feel something like what has been happening?

Looking carefully at what experience tells us can do more than helping us let go of strategies that are not working. They also can also provide a guide to what it is that we really want. That is why "creative hopelessness" is not actually "hopeless." It is "creative" because it is a kind of giving up that provides a key to help us go forward.

> Therapist: What if I were to say to you Elisabeth that maybe your sense of the hopelessness of this struggle are probably right. I don't mean that *you* are hopeless, but maybe all these strategies that you have been working so hard trying to eliminate pain and stress from your life may well be as hopeless as you are feeling right now.
>
> Elisabeth: You're not telling me that I will never get rid of my pain and feelings of burnout. I hope you're not saying that because I don't know how I could live if I can't get rid of the pain.
>
> Therapist: I don't need to tell you, Elisabeth You are the one with experience here in trying to get rid of your pain and stress feelings. What conclusions do you draw from the years and years and countless ways you have tried to eliminate pain and stress. Do you believe that it is possible to get rid of pain and stress from your life.
>
> Elisabeth: I really want to believe that, that is why I have worked so hard. I try to stay hopeful but, no, if I really look at the results of everything I have done, I would say no. I guess I knew in the back of my head, even when I came here to you that I would fail again. I just can't stand the thought of living with this pain and stress the rest of my life.
>
> Therapist: What if I were to say to you Elisabeth that in that hopelessness you are feeling right now that there is a very important value that could help you find a way.
>
> Elisabeth: What value, I don't see any way out.
>
> Therapist: Elisabeth. Why have you been fighting so hard to get rid of your pain and stress feelings, why didn't you just give up?
>
> Elisabeth: I fought because I wanted my life back. I want to work again, and play with my kids like I used to and sing again.

Therapist: That's exactly what I thought Elisabeth You fought because you valued something on the other side of that pain. The pain was what was in between you and something that you very much wanted, your life. If that had not been so, you would have given up long ago.

Elisabeth: How do I get there now, if I can't get rid of the pain?

Therapist: What if you could get there, Elisabeth How much would it be worth to you?

Elisabeth: You mean, if I could work again, be active in my family, get my friends back and all those things we talked about?

Therapist: Yes, Elisabeth I believe that getting your life back in the way that you want to live is very possible for you to do.

Elisabeth: That would be incredible. Of course, I would do about anything to get that.

Therapist: So, if I gave you a choice Elisabeth In one hand, I have a package where you would never have pain or stress again in your life. You could do this; it is entirely within your reach. But in this same package you do not get back your life. Because the cost of being painless and stressless is being literally knocked out by drugs. In the other package, you will have about the same amount of pain and stress as you do now, maybe more or less, but in this package you will get access to all those life areas you want to reclaim, your job, activities with your husband and family and friends and so on. Which package would you choose?

Elisabeth: Of course I would take the one with my life back but I don't think I can live with that pain.

Therapist: I didn't ask you if you thought you *could* do it, I just want to know if that is what *you want*, what you really want.

Elisabeth: Yes, of course it is!

Therapist: Ok. Then, that is what I want to work together with you doing in this therapy. I am on your team working with you to reclaim your life.

Elisabeth: That sounds good but how is that going to be possible?

At this point, in the "values first" approach we are following in this book, the clinician would probably move heavily into values exploration and clarification. However, in order to get a broader initial sense of how the chronic pain processes identified in the previous chapter are targeted in ACT it seems helpful to cover some of these methods at this point.

Targeting the Underlying Processes in Chronic Pain

The ACT model of intervention in pain is directly is linked to the model of chronic pain, as is shown in Figure 8.1. Instead of avoidance, acceptance; instead of fusion, defusion and mindfulness; instead of the domination of the conceptualized self and its seeming need for protection, a transcendent self of self is encouraged; instead of living in the past or future, richer contact with the present is encouraged; instead of vague or absent values, processes of values clarification; instead of waiting for life to start, committed action; and all of this in the service of a life richly, vitally, and flexibly lived.

A variety of content areas are likely to appear as barriers for the chronic pain patient. These include not just pain itself, but a much broad range of events such as cognition and emotion connected to history of failure; cognition regarding the certainty of future failure; a sense of not caring about anything; or client feelings of hopelessness. ACT therapists do not argue or try to deal with the content of barriers such as these however appealing or "true" they are. The issue is not literal but functional "truth."

Defusion and acceptance are implicit in every moment of interaction around barriers in ACT. These issues are steeped in the very fabric of dialogue in an ACT session.

> Therapist: I believe that reclaiming your life back is possible Elisabeth, but I need to know how much it would be worth to you. I need to know if you are willing to feel the pain and stress that you have been working so hard to avoid.
>
> Elisabeth: How in the world could I do that, this pain and feelings of stress is my enemy. It has ruined my life.
>
> Therapist: Exactly, and you have said that you don't want pain and stress to continue to ruin your life. You want your life back?
>
> Elisabeth: I don't see how I could have both. I have tried to control and manage pain and stress and live my life and it didn't work. I know it doesn't work.
>
> Therapist: Lets look at those statements. Give me an example of your experiences of failure.

(On white board)

Where were you going?	Stories	Led to?
Wanted to go to an evening course	I have tried before and failed	don't bother

> Therapist: So you saw an evening course in meditation that you wanted to go to, that was in your valued direction of spirituality and own leisure time interests, you thought about calling and getting registered, and then the thought came " I've tried before and failed, why bother, forget it" and that thought led to that you did not try.
>
> Elisabeth: That's right because I know that it just won't work, I can't sit that long.
>
> Therapist: Lets look at that statement

(On white board)

Where were you going?	Stories	Led to?
Meditation course	I know it won't work	didn't go
	I can't sit that long	

Elisabeth: But its true, I can't sit that long.

Therapist: Elisabeth Just look at what that statement led to. You were trying to do something for yourself that would lead you closer to reclaiming your life and when you went in that direction, this thought that you recognize came up and told you that you couldn't do it. It reminded you of past failures and warned you not to try. And at that point you listened to that thought and let it steer you off the course that you wanted to go. Was that thought your friend in the sense that you came closer to reclaiming your life?

Elisabeth: No but I do have that experience of failure.

Therapist: Let's look at a bus metaphor. We say that you are the bus driver and are using your compass to drive towards the teacher job that you really want to have. In your bus, you have a bunch of passengers which are your past experiences. We know that most of these passengers carry negative warnings about past failures. That most of our thoughts are negative alarms has to do with our "stone age" brain which functions to warn us about not getting eaten up by predators. While you are driving your bus towards new and challenging activities that you want to go, the passengers come up to you, sometimes one by one and sometimes all at the same time and make threats, warning you to turn off course and avoid all uncomfortable feelings or situations. They don't remind you of all of the many times you have succeeded and grown from your challenges in life. They only remind you of your failures and warn you to stop and avoid discomfort. There is, of course, "truth" to these stories that you have, in fact, had failures, but it is also true that you have much more experience of successes and this is not what shows up when you attempt to challenge yourself and take steps in valued directions. While you are driving towards your directions in reclaiming your life, these bus passengers are showing up, Elisabeth warning you of your past failures, and what have you been doing?

Elisabeth: I have been listening to them and doing what they tell me.

Therapist: Which means what?

Elisabeth: That I have been avoiding doing what I really want to do. These thoughts are so scary.

Therapist: We can get back to what is so scary about the passengers, but what have you been trying to do with them.

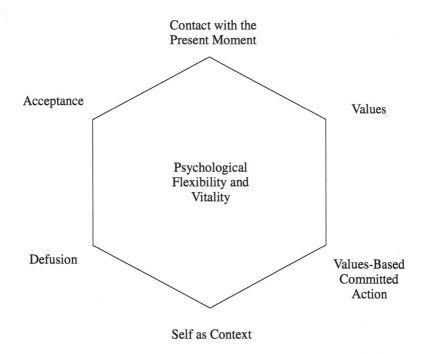

Figure 8.1. An ACT model of Intervention for Chronic Pain

Elisabeth: Reason with them, try to get rid of them, try to think positive thoughts to compete with them, try to drown them with pills.

Therapist: Has that worked, have you been able to reason with them or get rid of them?

Elisabeth: No, the more I reason with them the more they are on my mind and they never go away.

Therapist: Is this like the pain and stress? No matter how hard you try to get rid of it, it just stays there or gets worse.

Elisabeth: Yes, and while I have been on sick leave I have had more time to wrestle and reason with these thoughts but it seems like they have grown. Before I was out everyday working and going to town, now they even warn me about going out at all. How can I stop them?

Therapist: What if this is like the pain and stress, E? What if you cannot stop? You have tried and the more you try the bigger they get just like the pain and stress.

Elisabeth: What do I do then?

Therapist: The passengers on your bus are your past history, not all of your history but some of it. I don't know any way that human beings can remove their history, what is there, is there. But you can add on new history.

Elisabeth: You mean I can never get rid of those passengers, my negative thoughts.

Therapist: You can answer that yourself from you own experience. We cannot remove our thoughts but we can choose how we react to the thoughts and feelings. You can choose to listen to them and do what they tell you to or not.

Elisabeth: You mean I should ignore them?

Therapist: No, I mean you can acknowledge and accept them as thoughts and feelings from past history but that you choose to drive your bus forward into the discomfort that is necessary to step up to the challenges of going forward.

Elisabeth: Do you mean that I will have to risk pain and stress and failure. How do I know I will succeed? Can you guarantee me that if I went into pain and stress that I would succeed?

Therapist: No one can guarantee success Elisabeth. The question is, are you willing to take that risk, in order to give you self a chance for success. You may and probably will fail at times and succeed at times, but you will go forward closer to living the life you want.

Elisabeth: That sounds very scary but yes I am willing to take that chance.

Targeted Interventions

A wide variety of targeted ACT exercises and metaphors can also be used to transform barriers. These exercises are not ends in themselves. Rather, they are situated in a values context. For example an ACT therapist might use experiential exercises and homework to facilitate contact with avoided values, to disrupt ruminative self-punishment over past failures in valued domains; or to build greater flexibility with respect to avoided psychological content that emerges as barriers to pursuing values.

The client with longstanding pain and stress has established a history of avoidance strategies for the discomfort of pain, stress and many things that are associated with these aversive feelings. Exposure to pain, risk of pain and or feelings of stress will be difficult and is motivated by the client him/herself only it that it is a necessary threshold to cross to "reclaim" the life the client wants to live. Without the values context, exposure would be only "aversive". Without the context of values, the client may go through the motions of exposure but only to show compliance with the program that an insurance agency is demanding. Using the values context may insure that the client integrates the reasons for acceptance-based exposure as a vehicle to reclaim a valued life, rather than a way to please the rehabilitation staff or insurance companies. (See exposures exercises for past and future failing in Wilson & Luciano, 2002).

Dialogue with Elisabeth: Exposure to Failing

Therapist: What is it Elisabeth that is so scary, for example about your
    direction of going back to school?
Elisabeth: The thought that I would fail.
Therapist: Is fear of failing really what is keeping you from going forward
    to what you want and need to do?
Elisabeth: Yes, I am terrified of putting myself in a situation where I would
    fail at what I most want to do.
Therapist: Can you close your eyes Elisabeth and think about old examples
    of when you have experienced this terrible feeling of failing. Just try
    to feel that feeling of total failure and see what pictures come up for
    you. If a picture comes up, tell me about it.
Elisabeth: That's not hard, I remember a situation where I was about 15,
    and it was my last year in school. It was math class and we had a
    substitute teacher. I had gotten stuck in a problem and I somehow
    dared to raise my hand for help, which I didn't normally do. The
    teacher seemed kind of nervous and tried to answer very fast and I
    didn't understand what she meant and asked her again. She got mad
    at me and said very loud that I must be a very stupid girl if I can't even
    get what she was saying to me and that some people were just not
    meant to go on in school. (Meaning me). I was so embarrassed and sad
    I wanted to disappear threw the floor. If I hadn't cared about school so
    much it wouldn't have matter but she touched such a tender spot. I
    really wanted to go on with school. After that I gave up my dream.
Therapist: Stay with that feeling Elisabeth Where do you feel that bad
    feeling of failure and hopelessness.
Elisabeth: I feel in tightening in my chest and a queasy feeling in my
    stomach.
Therapist: And what are your thoughts and feelings?
Elisabeth: That I am a hopelessly stupid person. That it was so stupid of
    me to even think that I could get an education. That I should have
    listened to my family and just get a job and settle for a simpler easier
    life. That I would never again allow someone to say that to me or risk
    failing again. I would make sure I never failed.
Therapist: Do you recognize these thoughts and feelings from your bus
    passengers, the ones who come up to you when you are trying to go
    somewhere you want to go and tell you not to try.
Elisabeth: Yes, those are the scariest ones.
Therapist: What if I were to say Elisabeth you need to be willing to feel this
    awful feeling that you are feeling right now, and even other awful
    feelings in order to go on and reclaim your life. Would you be willing
    to feel them? Would it be worth it?

Elisabeth: You mean that I need to feel bad in order to feel good?

Therapist: I mean that in order to move towards those directions you want to go to like for example going back to school, you will be putting yourself in a situation where you risk failing. You may fail and you may not. The only way to guarantee no failing is what?

Elisabeth: Never to try.

Therapist: Right, same as the way to stay pain and stress free, avoid and stayed drugged.

Elisabeth: I have already said that I don't want to do that.

Therapist: So when you step up to the challenges of what you want to do, those bus passengers from the past are going to show up and warn you and when you continue to go forward you are taking risks and you may fail. You may also succeed and if you don't give yourself the chance you will never know.

Elisabeth: I would like to know that I would succeed before I dare do that.

Therapist: So would we all, but Elisabeth that is not life. We all have to be willing to look stupid, fail, and embarrass ourselves when we step up to a challenge.

Elisabeth: Ok I am willing to feel that to go forward.

Therapist: With the thought of your direction of education and going back to school. What could you do to go in that direction?

Elisabeth: I know what I could do, I have thought of it hundreds of times. I want to go to the Adult continuing education center in town and talk to them about how I could finish high school to be able to go on to the teacher's education.

Therapist: And what thought show up when you think of doing just that.

Elisabeth: Those same old passengers that say " you are stupid", "you are not the type of person that goes on to school", "you won't make it", "you are too old" you will look ridiculous ", and all of that.

Therapist: And how do you treat these passengers.

Elisabeth: I let myself feel them and I accept that they are there but I choose to go in the direction I want to go.

Therapist: That sounds great, Elisabeth But what if they are right and you do fail.

Elisabeth: Then I will try again because I want my life back.

Therapist: I am on your team E.

Acceptance-based exposure and defusion can include imaginal exercises, out of session assignments, interoceptive exposure, or exposure to overt situations. For example, Gutiérrez et al. (2004) developed a clever variant of the ACT "cards exercise" (Hayes et al., 1999, p. 162) for pain. Participants were asked to write pain-related thoughts that had previously lead to task avoidance (e.g. "I can't stand this pain.") cards. These were put aside and they were given a folded piece of paper and asked to imagine that the folded paper that had just been given contained one of the thoughts. They then were asked to stand up and move through the room carrying the paper, finally sitting and down reading it for the first time. The sentence on the piece of paper was: "I can't stand up." This experience then structured a discussion of whether it is possible to have the pain related thoughts without avoidance: e.g., "Can you think 'I can't stand this pain' and then continue with a painful task?"

Similarly, it has been shown that common ACT defusion and acceptance exercises such as the "leaves on a stream" (Hayes et al., 1999, 158-162) and "physicalizing" (Hayes et al., 1999, 170-171) can helpful in dealing effectively with pain (Takahashi, Muto, Tada, & Sugiyama, 2002). These exercises help teach the client how to observe thoughts and feelings without entanglement. Because these exercises (and scores of other ACT exercises like them) are so readily modifiable to the topic of pain, the ACT clinician working with pain clients has a rich palette of clinical tasks readily at hand.

Self as Context

It is helpful to support the client, as they learn defusion and acceptance techniques, in finding a safe, humane place from with exposure can be done. Mindfulness and acceptance leads naturally to a transcendent sense of self as the client starts to disidentify themselves with their own thoughts and feelings. This following exercise is adapted to the application of pain from a stress-focused version (Bond & Hayes, 2002).

> Close your eyes Elisabeth and follow my voice. I want you to take a deep breath and slowly exhale. Imagine that when you are breathing in, you take in all your body needs and when you slowly exhale you let go of everything your body does not need. Imagine that the air is breathing you; you can just let go and relax. You will be "breathed" without any effort on your part, just let go and relax. Now. Picture yourself in this room, notice any sounds in the room, or outside of the room. Notice any emotions you are having, Notice any thoughts that you are having. Now, get in touch with the "observer", the part of you that has noticed the bodily sensation, the feelings, the thoughts. This is the part of you that has always been you and will always be you. The you that knows about those values that have always been and will always be constant in your life. As the observer listen and follow these thoughts:
>
> My body is constantly changing. My body may find itself in different conditions of health or sickness, in a painful or stressful condition. It may be rested or tired, weak or strong. My body started out as a baby and grew continuously, and will continue to change and gradually grow old. Through my life experiences I will hurt myself and get scarred. I may loose a part of my body. My body can become fat or thin. My muscles can become stiff and weak or flexible and strong. Yet through all of this the part of me that

is observing my body has been constant. I have been me my whole life. Thus, I have a body, yet I don't experience that I am my body. When my body changes, I am still me. Focus your attention on this central concept. Allow yourself to realize this as your experience, not just a thought. Think of all the ways your body has changed throughout your lifetime, while you, Elisabeth remained constant." Sometimes, Elisabeth, you may forget that you are not your body and you might think, "I am a person with pain" or " I am a stress sensitive person". Return to the observer Elisabeth and see that pain and stress are feelings that come and go and constantly change while you Elisabeth remain constant and can observe this changes.
(short silence)

Now, consider this: I have different roles to play, and yet I am not these roles. My roles are many and constantly changing. Sometimes I'm in the role of a worker at my job, and sometimes, I am in my role as a mother, and a housewife and a lover. Sometimes I am in the role of a friend and sometimes the role of a student. I play some role all of the time. If I were to try and not play a role, I would be playing that role of not playing a role. Even now as I sit here, I am playing a role of a client sitting with a therapist. Yet, all the while, the observer, the part of me I call "I" or Elisabeth is watching. I can play my constantly changing roles, yet all the while, I can be there as a constant, steady observer of it all. So, again, I have roles, I play roles constantly, but I am not my roles. Allow yourself to realize that you have experienced this and continue to experience this. Sometimes, you forget this and have thoughts that you are your roles. You might have thoughts Elisabeth that you are the role of a patient with fibromyalgia. Return to the observing Elisabeth and see this role as just one of the many roles you have played in your lifetime. Roles that are constantly changing and will continue to constantly change while you Elisabeth remain constant with your values.

Now, keep the position as the observing Elisabeth and consider this: I have many emotions. My emotions are countless, contradictory, and changing constantly. They may swing from love to hatred, calm to anger, stressed to relaxed, pain to no pain, and yet I, Elisabeth with my constant values have been here, through all of these changes and contradictions. I can feel both love and hatred towards my family within minutes of each other, yet my constant value of maintaining close and loving relationships in my family remains constant. I can feel hopeful and hopelessness in the situation of education, while my value of continuing in education remains constant. I can feel excitement and anger and pain at my work place and employer while my value of having an employment in my life remains constant. I can feel the pulsating joy of a physical workout and the awful pain of sore muscles while I maintain the value of good physical fitness. Even now, I am experiencing... interest, boredom, embarrassment, relaxation. And, throughout, I am capable of observing it all and maintaining my constant values. Though a wave of emotion may come over me, it will pass in time. The observer part of me knows that I am having this emotion and yet I *am not* this emotion. The emotions that I experience are constantly changing, but the observer Elisabeth remains constant through it all, noticing the changes; thus I have emotions but I am not my emotions. Focus on this concept: I have emotions but I am not my emotions. Sometimes, Elisabeth you may forget this and have thoughts that you are your emotions. You might think, your feelings of anger and pain about your workplace are really true and will always be there. But the observer Elisabeth has seen these feelings of anger and pain in many situations and knows that feelings like this come and go as they always have and always will while you Elisabeth remain constant together with your values. The observer Elisabeth knows that emotions are constantly changing."

Finally, let's turn to what may be the most difficult area; your own thoughts. Consider this, I have thoughts, but I am not my thoughts. My thoughts are constantly changing. In my life, I have gained new ideas, new knowledge, and new experiences. I could have had a strong opinion or idea about something to be true and later find out this to be false. I could have thought something to be false and then found out it to be true and totally different than what I thought. Sometimes my thoughts are very childish or foolish and don't make sense at all. Sometimes my thoughts just appear automatically, like out of nowhere for no apparent reason. The observer Elisabeth knows that I have these thoughts, yet I am not these thoughts. You, Elisabeth had thoughts that showed up when you were about to go into the meeting and talk about how to start your education. Thoughts showed up like " who do you think you are?" "you are too old" "you are too stupid to get an education". These thoughts just showed up. Let the observer Elisabeth just observe these thoughts without getting caught up in them. Just let them show up and notice that they are constantly changing in countless, sometimes contradictory forms. Just let them flow and return to your position of observer. You observe these thoughts and recognize them because they come up in many situations but you are not these thoughts, you, Elisabeth, remain constant and with your valued directions in life watching it all flow. So now, watch your thoughts for a few moments and see what happens when you just watch your thoughts as they pass by you as a stream.

Notice what is left with you, you and the valued directions you have in life which you always have had and always will have regardless of the changes in your body, your roles your feelings or your thoughts that pass by. You are not just your body, your roles, feelings or thoughts. Those things are the content of your life, while you and your values are the arena, the context, and the space in which they unfold. As you see that, notice how you can distance yourself from the things you have been struggling with and putting up with. You, Elisabeth have been trying to change your roles, your feelings, you have been trying to get rid of "bad" feelings of stress and pain, trying to control your mind and bodily reactions. And the more you have tried, the worse it gets, the more entangled you become, the less YOU are even there. You've been trying to change the content in you life, but you don't have to change your roles, thoughts, feelings or body or memories before your life can work they way you want it to work because these things are not you anyway. They will come and go in your life just as they always have, why struggle with them? Why not, Elisabeth, focus on your constant values, your life compass, and do the things right now, that are consistent with your valued directions. Do the things that will help you achieve the goals and dreams that are consistent with the life you value.".?

Now, again, picture yourself in this room, and now picture the room (the room is described), and when you are ready to come back into the room, open your eyes. What was your experience of this exercise, Elisabeth? What were the things you tried to avoid here"?

This exercise helps establish a sense of the client as distinct from the psychological content that is being struggled with. Normal humans are conscious, verbal beings. By connecting with that sense of continuity of consciousness it is more possible to open to feared events, without a sense of imminent self-destruction.

Contacting the Present Moment

Life does not go on in the past or future. It only occurs now. Yet language itself disguises this simple fact. Pain clients who are drawn into a struggle with pain put their life on hold, living instead for the future in which pain will diminish and life can begin again. Meantime the clock continues to tick. Children grow up. Careers progress or deteriorate.

Any method that reorients the client toward now, as it is experienced directly to be, will increase vitality and flexibility. Becoming more mindful of simple tasks, noticing what is in the immediate environment more flexibly, or learning to watch thoughts come and go are all examples.

ACT is intellectually allied with mindfulness approaches of all kind, some of which have been applied to chronic pain. ACT can readily accommodate such methods as mindfulness meditation (Kabat-Zinn, 1990), or "just noticing" thoughts and feelings while engaging in daily tasks.

From an ACT perspective the four left-most processes of the hexagon in Figure 8.1 define what mindfulness is at the level of process. Each is facilitative of the other. Contacting the present moment only leads to mindfulness if it is non-judgmental, which is facilitated by defusion from evaluative and temporal relational frames and by acceptance of the experiences that arise. All of this is facilitated by a sense of self as the conscious context for experiences, rather than as the content of those experienced.

In one sense, ACT as a whole is an "informal practice" of mindfulness and meditation. Formal practice, such as following the breath, can facilitate the skills that informal practice requires. But it is informal practice – the walking meditation called "life" – that is ultimately most important for clinical progress.

Values

We return now to the issue of values, which provides the meaningful context for all of this work. From an ACT perspective clients "get stuck" while spending more and more time trying to control, manage or alleviate pain and stress symptoms while less and less time is being spent acting in valuable life directions. The symptoms of pain and stress begin to occupy the client's life and valuable time and energy is used to take care of the symptoms rather than live in a way is meaningful. Valued life domains get put on hold while energy is spent revolving around futile efforts to eliminate that cannot be eliminated. In this respect, the client who is "stuck" in pain/ stress symptoms has a values imbalance, or even what might be thought of as a kind of values illness. This is the reason in the present approach we have emphasized that the client's values should be identified from the start and all through therapy and follow-up as the reference from which therapy is framed. The core treatment strategy is defused and accepting exposure to the pain and stress which they client has been avoiding, consciously and in the moment, but all of this is done in the context of the client's valued directions.

In the case of Elisabeth, she said she came into therapy "because I suffer from unbearable pain and I can't tolerate any stress or demands on me." She believed that she had these symptoms "because I have taken too much responsibility, at work, at home, everything just got too much and overwhelmed me. My workload has gotten more and more demanding and I got stressed out overworked." She sought to solve this problem in this way: "I have generally rested and avoided everything that I think causes me to feel stressed and pain. I have really tried to listen to my feelings and take care of myself for the first time in my life." Her goals of therapy were "I hope you can help me to manage the stress and pain better so that I can be a little less handicapped."

This was Elisabeth's life compass (Figure 8.2). Once constructed it can be pre-printed for therapy sessions or can be drawn on a whiteboard and done together with the client.

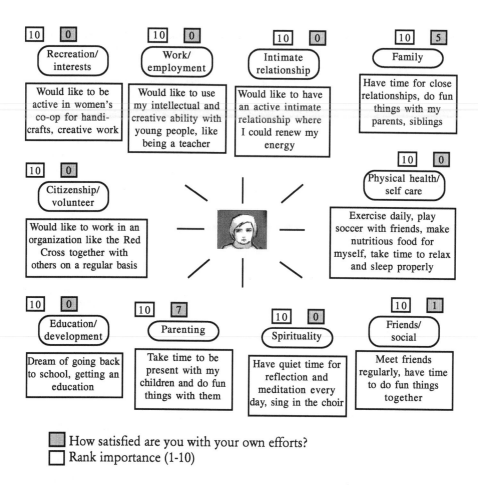

Figure 8.2. Elisabeth's Life Compass.

To look at Elisabeth life history, there is a pattern of "taking care of others" which has had highest priority and "taking care of oneself" in any significant way that has had lowest priority. Until the time where Elisabeth went on sick leave she, spent all her time and energy at her job, caretaking, with her family and relatives, caretaking. Very little time was spent in activities such as preventive health, education, developing own interests and social life that have been shown to "protect" against developing chronic illness. After Elisabeth went on sick leave and long-term disability leave she experienced nearly complete losses in life quality in 8 of 10 life domains (discrepancy of 10). It should not be a surprise that she feels depressed and hopeless about her life situation. Any domain showing significant discrepancy is a target for start of treatment. The question for the clinician is "why aren't the client's feet going in that direction?"

Clients with longstanding pain/stress will often show obsessive thinking with a focus on symptom alleviation and have difficulty with thinking in terms of long-term goals. They will make such statements as: "It is a full time job these days to take care of myself, let alone think of working;" "I would be happy if I could just be pain-free a few minutes a day"; "Some day, researcher will find a cure for my pain, but for right now I just need to make sure I avoid making it worse"; or "I know now what causes my pain and stress, and I work very hard avoiding those things."

Doing the VLQ in the first session can help the client see beyond short-term symptom alleviation. The tone of the work is important. Here is an example of how this part of therapy sounds.

Dialogue with Elisabeth and Therapist:

Elisabeth: I want you to think about these values in terms of long-term directions that have been pretty constant in your life. Like the importance of education, work and having friends in your life.

Elisabeth: Why should I do that, it hurts to do that. I know I will never be able to live up to that, why should I even think about them. I've accepted the fact that I will never have those things again. I've accepted that I am sick. I have a diagnosis. It is a full time job just to take care of myself. I don't want to think about those things.

Therapist: I am not asking you what is realistic; I am asking you what you value and what your life would look like in the best of all worlds.

Elisabeth: Why should I do that, it hurts to think of it.

Therapist: Ok, lets take an example from education. You wrote that you valued education at 10 and then you wrote that you had a zero for your own activities towards the education you would like. What were you thinking?

Elisabeth: When I was a little girl, up to the age of 10 I dreamed about getting an education and being a teacher. I was very good in school and I liked school. But my brothers who were ahead of me really hated school and gave the teachers a hard time and dropped out early. I felt that my teachers didn't expect much from me and my family just laughed at my ideas of an education. They wanted me to quit school early and get a job. At some point I figured they were right and gave up the idea, but I did have that dream.

Therapist: Elisabeth I want you to close your eyes and find a picture of that little girl, 10 years old, sitting at her desk, bright eyed and curious about learning. Do you see her? I want you to feel that dream about getting an education and wanting to be a teacher. Can you feel what she is feeling and dreaming about?

Elisabeth: Yes she is thinking about all the books she could read and the type of teacher she would like to be.

Therapist: Elisabeth would you give this little girl a second chance to realize this dream if you could?

Elisabeth: Of course I would.

Therapist: Even if it cost you pain and hard work, would you still be willing to give this little girl a chance to reach her dream.

Elisabeth: Yes, of course I would. I would do about anything to give her that chance.

Therapist: Open your eyes Elisabeth that's how I want you to think about that value and the rest of them. It does hurt to see that you haven't given yourself the chance to realize what you dream of but if you are willing to feel that hurt, you would give yourself a chance of getting closer. If not for yourself, think of that little girl, or the role model you are for your own children, as you deny yourself the possibility of realizing a dream.

Elisabeth: That's true, I want my own children to be the best they can be, and even my old friends, but I settle for less.

Therapist: Yes, if you look at your life compass, you have compromised important values in the service of pain/stress management.

It is helpful to identify life values compass by using the VLQ in all domains before continuing. Covering all domains is worthwhile precisely because chronic pain tends to narrow repertoires and human lives. By pushing for a broad view of what is meaningful a more flexible set of actions are available to motivate and sustain change.

Values are not something that be achieved like an object; or achieved in the future. They are instantiated moment by moment in a continuous never-ending process of living itself. The VLQ asked clients to rate 1) importance, 2) intentions, and 3) consistency of activities relative to valued intentions. All three are important to keep the focus properly on continuous behavior in the moment – values should be described as unreachable but continuously present directions rather than goals that can be completed.

Returning to the life compass we ask client about the directions of their own activities. Referring to the compass, we ask in what direction the client's feet are going, towards or away from the valued directions (intentions).

A line can be drawn from the person in the middle of the compass out towards each valued direction and the question asked "Do your feet go towards your intention?" The answer is usually "no," followed by a number of "stories" given, which usually revolve around the symptom. For example:

Stories: "I don't have time"
             "I don't have the energy"
             "There are more important things I must do"
             " I'm no longer interested".

" A person with pain can't do those things"
" I am sensitive to stress".
" I can't tolerate any demands".

These "stories" should be written down together with the client. This exercise illustrates 1) that the client's feet are mostly not going in directions consistent with valued life directions, and 2) there are patterns or themes in the stories given as to why feet are not moving in valued directions. Themes typically focus on giving priority to "taking care" of the symptom. Compromises shown in the form of moving in directions inconsistent with valued directions are "excused" with taking care of symptoms. Defusion and acceptance skills need to be applied at that point to the reasons the client's mind provided for a failure to live in a vital way.

Dialogue with Elisabeth

Therapist: When you look at the figures you've given on your life compass, what do you see?

Elisabeth: I see that I am far from living the life that I at one time want to live, but I have accepted that now. I am really not interested in much of any of those things; I just try and make it through the day, with as little pain as possible.

Therapist: I can see that you have experienced major losses in 8 of 10 life domains. These are significant losses. Why couldn't you, for example, reclaim your friendships and get that back in your life the way you would like it to be.

Elisabeth: That is just not possible, because of the pain and stress it would be. I know I just can't do it. I don't really care anyway.

Therapist: But you wrote that you do care, that you would like to have close friends in your life, that a sense of community is something you have always valued.

Elisabeth: Yes, I said that, but I can't have it. Taking care of everything I have   to do plus taking care to avoid pain and stress is a full time job. That   was just a dream.

Therapist: Lets write these obstacles that are getting in the way between you and where you would like to be going on the boards. Let's call them "stories". I'll write here "stories" and a big BUT and then next to this heading I'll write "leads to".

Elisabeth: Ok, but they are not stories that I have made up, it is true that I have pain and have become very sensitive to demands and all stress. I was told to be very careful and listen to my body.

Therapist: I'm not evaluating if these "stories" are true or not, or even if they are probable, I just want to write down the reasons or statements that you say to yourself that seem to steer your feet in another direction than the way you want to be going. Is that ok? Now, lets keep going. What about the intention you gave about wanting an active intimate relationship. What are the reasons you have for not putting your feet in that direction and creating the relationship you want?

Elisabeth: That's easy, because of my pain. Its hurts to move and my husband is pretty insensitive. Besides I don't think he is interested. I've gained weight besides and I don't think he would find me attractive any more.

Therapist: Lets write these "stories" down.

It is important never to argue or engage in the content of these statements but think instead in terms of function. What does saying these statements lead to? How do the statements serve the client?

Such an analysis might lead to a picture such as this:

Intention	Stories BUT	leads to
Social Would like to call old friend	cannot sit due to pain	don't call
Intimate Would like to tell my husband how I would like to be touched	he wouldn't be interested	don't try
Work Would like to visit work	I would feel anxious, pain	don't try
Health Would like to play soccer	It would be painful, embarrassing	don't try
Education Would like to go back to school	could not sit long time	don't try
Spiritual Would like to sing in the choir	would be demanding and stressful	stay home

Dialogue with Elisabeth

Therapist: Elisabeth do these "stories" have anything in common?

Elisabeth: Yes, there are similar but they are true just the same, I have experienced all those feelings.

Therapist: I didn't ask you Elisabeth if they were true, I just wondered if what they had in common. How they serve you.

Elisabeth: The stories are mostly about avoiding my pain, and they led to me not trying.

Therapist: Its looks like you had a pretty good idea of where you wanted to go, but when you started off in that direction, these uncomfortable thoughts or feelings would show up, mostly warning you about how you might feel, and they steered you off course, I mean in another direction than you intended to go.

Elisabeth: Yes but, those thoughts and feelings are usually right, I have experienced pain in those situations.

Therapist: Let me give you an example Elisabeth of what I mean. Tonight is my aerobics night at the gym. I know from many years of experience that I come closer to my health directions when I go to this workout class. I build up my muscles, I can relax better, I sleep better, I am nicer to my family and I am more alert at work if I go regularly to gymnastics. I know all this. But when I come home, I just don't *feel* like going. My "story" I say to myself is "I am just too tired" "I have worked all day, I deserve, a break", "I'll go next time". What those stories lead to is that I stay home. Staying home, gives me some immediate relief of not having to get up and go out, but what does it do in the long run.

Elisabeth: Make you more tired?

Therapist: Yes and makes it harder for me to go next time. You could say that on the one hand I had my experience telling me: go to the workout, even if it's tough, you will get closer to the physical fitness you want and on the other hand, I had feelings and thoughts in the form of "stories" that were telling me to avoid the stress and strain of going out again and just stay home. Who is my friend here, who is steering me in my valued direction of working towards a long-term better health?

Elisabeth: Your experience.

Therapist: Right, my experience tells me that getting over that short threshold of uncomfortablness would bring me closer to where I myself wanted to go, but my feelings and thoughts were telling me the opposite, to give in to feelings of discomfort and stay comfortable. Should feelings be trusted?

Elisabeth: Maybe not, maybe my own experience is what I should be listening to.

Therapist: If you look back at your life compass and the stories you wrote as obstacles, in what directions have you been steered?

Elisabeth: But this is what the Health Care professionals told me to do. Avoid stress and pain, listen to my body. Rest and don't exert yourself. Take pain-killers, don't do anything that hurts or that causes stress.

Therapist: Let's make a list of those attempts you have experienced to solve pain and stress. What you have tried and what it had led to. First I must ask you Elisabeth how do you think you will ever closer to those intentions.

Elisabeth: By first getting rid of the pain and living a less stressful life. The day I feel better I will try and reclaim my life.

Therapist: Lets look at the ways you have tried to do just that. We can look at ways which you have tried and try to both prevent pain and stress and also once you have it, how you try to control or manage pain/stress. We can look first at what kind of strategies you use and we can look at the results you get in the short term and in the long term relative to where you want to be going.

Choosing which areas of life domains to start with in therapy requires good clinical judgment. Larger discrepancies in the VLQ can be a guide. For example, Elisabeth holds a constant value that education is important (10) but she has made no effort at all (feet) in the direction during the past week (0). She shows the maximal discrepancy in this domain. Since Elisabeth has a difference of 10 in many other domains as well, however, this rule is ambiguous. Another approach is to consider how these domains relate to each other. For example, getting the type of job that Elisabeth wants will depend on Elisabeth going back to school. Therefore, activities towards an education might be a wise first step.

Problem:	Tips
What therapy goal to choose	Look at areas with significant discrepancies
	Emphasize importance of all areas & let client see what shows up
	Is one area holding up other areas? If so, consider focusing on earlier steps
	In one area more likely to move quickly? If so, consider this area.
Clients may feel stressed that they must live up to living directions.	Introduce the idea of quality rather than quantity in activities: being in the bull's eye.
	Emphasize process, not outcome
	Mindfulness training in feeling vitality in an activity.

> Discrimination training in what feels vital and what others what you to do.
>
> Discuss the idea of balance and vitality in all valued directions rather than using values as a form of negative judgment

Concrete goals can be useful temporarily provided they cohere with values. Often with traditional cognitive behavior therapy, we have learned to use quantifiable objective goals and to break these goals down in small measurable steps. There is nothing wrong with this approach per se but it can miss the importance of the larger directions that make these specific goals meaningful.

Thus, in addition to tracking steps towards specific goals it is helpful to focus on whether the client is in alignment with the valued direction. There is a natural feedback that comes from moving in a valued direction: a sense of flexibility and vitality. Over time clients can sense whether they are moving in a valued direction. For example, consider a person who values being close to other people. This cannot be measured by the frequency of overt behaviors alone. Like an arrow that has "hit the mark" there is a sense of being in the bull's eye. A person who is going on a walk with a friend will sense whether or not they are headed toward their value by a sense of openness, vulnerability, and sharing.

The goal in ACT is that all of the life domains viewed as important by the clients are alive and vital with activities that hitting the bull's eye. The activity could be large or small but it should be on target.

Conclusion

The ACT model of intervention contains several specific domains of intervention. It is not a specific protocol, nor a specific set of interventions. Just as traditional CBT concepts can support the development of myriad specific protocols, so too an ACT model can be adjusted to fit a variety of treatment settings, modes of intervention, types of difficulty, and sequence of components. As steps are taken toward a valued direction, barriers are inevitably encountered. Clients are challenged by two separate cycles (Hayes & Smith, in press).[1] As is shown in Figure 8.3 clients have a choice: to spiral upward in an acceptance cycle or downward in a control and avoidance cycle. The present volume is designed to show the nature of those two cycles in chronic pain and to empower clinicians to help clients consistently to choose the acceptance cycle. Doing so is personally challenging to therapists, however, a topic to which we now turn.

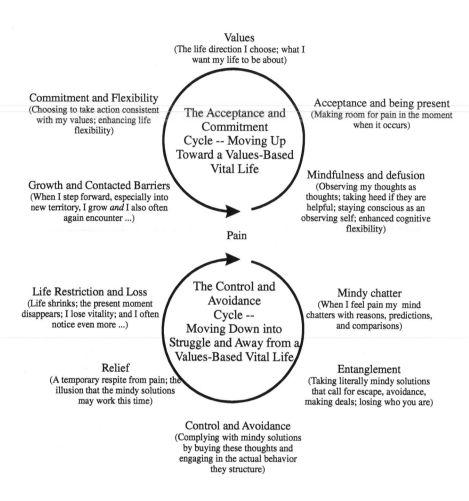

Figure 8.3. The two cycles pain clients can choose. The choice at the top cycles upward toward vitality, the choice at the at the bottom cycles downward into struggle. Note that both cycles involve repeated, perhaps even frequent, contact with pain. Adopted from an idea by David Chantry and modified by Hayes and Smith (in press).

Chapter 9

ACT for Therapists and Staff

"I don't think my therapist likes me or understands me. He is an educated person and seems nice but he lives in another world. At first he was kind and seemed to listen. But after awhile I could tell that he lost interest. I probably bored him. You can tell when someone is not listening by the look in his or her eyes. I figured that I must really be a hopeless case if this therapist who is supposed to be good in helping people can't help me."

Therapist Burnout

From an ACT perspective, care providers and even systems of care providers suffer from the same "problem" that plague our clients. Therefore, it is important to look at providers with the same lens. As suggested in the original ACT book (Hayes et al., 1999) personal work can help the therapist in several ways. First, the therapist can become sensitized to ways in which experiential avoidance negatively impacts their own work. A sensitivity to one's own experiential avoidance can be prescriptive. It can orient the therapist towards defusion and acceptance activities that can give them more flexibility in working with their clients and co-workers. Second, exposure, defusion and values work can be very challenging. Therapist' *personal* contact with this difficulty can eliminate some of the one-up/one-down quality that can endanger a therapeutic relationship. ACT therapists who have a sense that we are all in the same boat may be better prepared to act with compassion and to act more effectively when they share a sense of the magnitude of the task.

Questioning your Own Activities

One way to begin this sort of self assessment as a therapist is to ask a set of questions of yourself. Some of these questions will not apply to you as a therapist, while others may apply very directly. Why do you want to work with persons who are stuck in chronic pain or stress symptoms? How does it feel when you work very hard with a client who doesn't respond, or who responds only a short while and then goes back to old destructive behavior? Do you find yourself arguing with clients or trying hard to persuade them? How your feel when clients don't do the homework exercises you have put effort into creating? When you are unable to get a client moving, do you ever feel incompetent as a therapist? What do you do when you encounter feelings of incompetence, disappointment, and frustration?

Therapists confronted with refractory clients may engage in all manner of avoidance themselves in order to reduce feelings of incompetence or powerlessness.

They make take on the role of the expert and talk about studies and statistics. They may retreat, get sad, go to courses, read books, get sympathy from others. While not problematic in and of themselves, all these activities may serve the function of reducing the "bad" feelings that occur when you feel stuck as a therapist. The ACT therapist needs to examine how these things affect interactions with clients?

The effects of avoiding reactions to difficult clients can also easily spill over into our interactions with our colleagues. Consider times when you argued with your colleagues who had different ideas about the way therapy should be done or defended your work with a client even when it was not particularly effective. Does the sense of being stuck with your own clients generate inflexibility in your professional activities? Do you find yourself working to explain your treatment decisions or defend negative client outcomes? When you feel yourself trapped, frustrated, confused, afraid, angry or anxious, be glad. You are now in the same boat as the client, and that can inform and humanize your work.

Allowing yourself to feel and accept these negative feelings about yourself and your work may be the first step in becoming a better therapist. Your own pain, frustration, and feelings of incompetence may be an important point of entry in getting into contact with your client. Being compassionate with others may begin with being compassionate with yourself. Being willing to feel these "bad" feelings you have about yourself, without doing anything to reduce them, *and* while remaining committed to the work you chose, may make you a true fellow traveler with the clients you wish to serve.

Connecting to other Human Beings: What is that?

Most of us became therapists for the simple reason that we felt compassion for others and wanted to be of service to our fellow human beings. We get an education as a clinical psychologist, physician, physical or occupational therapist, nurse or social worker. We study for years about the workings of brain and body. We study theories, diagnoses, and treatment methods. We start working with clients after years of study, only to find out that there is an enormous difference between being knowledgeable about theories and being able to interact effectively with clients. All of us have read that the therapeutic alliance is an important component in all therapy forms, but few of us have ever learned specifically how to achieve that. After a year or two of working with clients, many become disillusioned. Our compassion seems to run low. Many clients do not get better at all, and those who do are not always thankful for our help. We start to doubt that we are such great therapists—a terrifying notion. We may create stories about what is wrong. Maybe we have the wrong diagnosis for the client. Maybe the client is hopeless. Maybe the client just wasn't motivated. The years pass and we, the therapists, may start to have stress symptoms ourselves. Headaches, backaches, and tense muscles are common among those who work as caregivers.

Opening up to Frustration, Uncertainty, and Feelings of Failure

The challenge for the ACT therapist is to create a context for thoroughgoing unconditional acceptance of feelings and thoughts of both you and your client. Some recent data suggest that feelings of stress and burnout are may be more a result of trying to manage and control these feelings than from the feelings themselves. In a recent study, drug counselors showed decreases in burnout and increases in sense of accomplishment with clients. Paradoxically, this lessening of burnout and increase in sense of accomplishment emerged from a training workshop that emphasized acceptance and openness to thoughts and feelings associated with burnout (Hayes, et al., 2004). Recognizing the ways our own thoughts, feelings and fears constrict our abilities to communicate with our clients and with our peers can facilitate the development of a potent therapeutic relationship.

The Therapist: Reclaiming Compassion

What should a therapist do who feels "burned-out" from working with chronic pain clients? Within an ACT model that question has special relevance since ACT can be used to reclaim the ingredients needed to be the therapists we want to be with chronic pain patients. From an ACT perspective, the barriers to working with chronic pain patients themselves provide important information about how humans function: both therapists and clients.

In order to show how the model applies we will walk through a dialogue between two clinical psychologists, stopping periodically to describe how the ACT model fits. One of the providers has felt increasing stress and burnout symptoms that he believes are caused by many years of working with refractory chronic pain patients. The second provider is a colleague well versed in the ACT model. In the scenario, the burned out therapist has come to his colleague to consult on the difficulty with burnout they are experiencing.

Burned out therapist (BOT): I have been thinking about getting out of rehabilitation. I just don't have it anymore. I spend most of the time mad. Mad at work. Mad at my clients. When I am not mad, I just feel exhausted. I just feel like I have to get out. I am sure not the therapist I planned to be.

ACT consultant (ACT-C): Sounds like a hard place to arrive.

BOT: Yes. Some days I feel very sad about it. Like I lost something important. I try to dig back in, find that spark, but nothing ever really lasts. I guess I just have to get out.

ACT-C: Well, there are two sorts of consultation I could provide. One sort is not terribly personal. Like if you came to me saying that you were sick of your car and all of the problems it had, I would tell you to sell it and I would tell you about two or three models that might make a good replacement. This seems like a different situation though. More like giving up on a family member or a marriage than like giving up

on a car. It sounds like it pulls at you–like there is something
personally painful about the idea of leaving.

BOT: Yes. I mean, I don't even know why it is so hard for me. It's not like
I couldn't get another job.

ACT-C: Right. That's what I was noticing. It seems like there is something
in this struggle that is of importance to you–more important than a mere
job change.

BOT: Yes, I think I see what you mean.

ACT-C: So one thing I could do is to talk to you about an exit strategy from
rehab, or maybe a couple strategies to make work more palatable. But,
my guess is that you have gone over that sort of thing yourself a million
times yourself. There is another sort of consult I could do though. This
other is more personal. It ends up being as much about you as about
the work. It would involve digging into the meaning of the work *for you*
as much as it involves the work itself. Emotionally, this conversation
would be more like talking about whether to have children or not than
it would be like deciding which type of car to buy. It is an Acceptance
and Commitment Therapy model of consultation. This model of
consulting looks more at how your work fits into your life and you in
into your work. I ask because I sense how meaningful this is to you. I
also ask because it is more personal, and likely more painful, and I
would not want to intrude without permission.

BOT: It's OK, really. I am at the end of my rope with this. Go ahead and
ask whatever you want. If it could help, it would be worth it.

This component of the consultation is the equivalent of informed consent in
a therapeutic interaction. When a colleague seeks guidance in a professional matter,
and the dominant model of consulting is largely didactic, we need to as clearly as
possible to make engagement in the consultation an informed choice. More
generally, just as in treatment, when we are about to orient a client to difficult work,
we ask permission to do so. Burdens undertaken by choice tend to be a bit lighter
than those imposed upon us (see Wilson & Murrell, 2004, for extended discussion
of the scientific basis of this claim).

ACT-C: OK. It starts with a pretty simple question: If you could chose,
what kind of a therapist would you chose to be?

BOT: A good therapist. One who helps people.

ACT-C: Is that the kind of therapist you are today?

BOT: Not at all. Well, I guess that is an exaggeration; but, I used to be
better. I don't know why. I just don't like my clients. I have heard so
many client stories that I am tired of them. Maybe I never was a good
therapist. Maybe I should go into teaching and research instead.

ACT-C: Why did you want to become a therapist?

BOT: I always like working with people and I dreamed about being useful to people who had problems. I thought I could make a difference in people's lives. I know it sounds sort of naïve.

ACT-C: And you don't value that anymore?

BOT: Of course I do, but now I am just more realistic. After years of working, I am not so hopeful anymore. I mean, clients mostly want someone to tell their stories to, and they really don't want to do anything about their problem.

ACT-C: And, if the thought that clients do not want to change could advise you, what advice would it give?

BOT: It would tell me to just sit back and let them tell their stories, give them the standard homework assignments and targets, and move on to the next client.

ACT-C: Would that thought tell you to invest yourself thoroughly in the client?

BOT: Well, I care about them.

ACT-C: Yes, but imagine the thought—'they don't really want to do anything'—could speak to you. Would it tell you to lean forward in your chair—invest yourself thoroughly?

BOT: Not really, no.

ACT-C: So the thought would tell you to lay back, listen a bit, then provide a pretty standard set of responses.

BOT: Yes.

ACT-C: And, if you asked that thought about its motives, wouldn't it say that it was trying to help you? Something like: 'Just take it easy. Not much is going to happen anyway, so don't spend too much of yourself in here. You'll just wear yourself out—and for no particular good reason.' Like a friend saying 'Hey, no use pounding your head against a wall.'

BOT: Well, that's how I feel.

ACT-C: Right, but if that thought could talk, is that how it would treat you. Maybe it would put its arm around your shoulder—give you a little pat on the back.

BOT: Sure.

ACT-C: And how would you feel toward that thought—imagining that it is a person? Does it feel like your friend?

BOT: Well, maybe like a friend that is telling me some hard fact, but trying to help. So, I sit back and let my clients tell their stories and don't have much ambition anymore. I am just being realistic. People don't really want to change. Mostly, they want to complain. So I let them complain and they pay me to sit and listen.

ACT-C: And that thought right there: 'I'm just being realistic.' If that thought could speak to you, what would it say? What advice would it give?

BOT: Pretty much to do what I am doing.

ACT-C: And the other one I noticed in there: 'People don't really want to change.'

BOT: The same.

ACT-C: If those thoughts were like a little advisory council—your own little personal committee of advisors—who would be the chair of the committee?

BOT: What?

ACT-C: You know if each one of those thoughts: 'they don't want to do anything,' 'I'm just being realistic,' 'they don't want to change' were all like a room full of people, helping you decide what to do—who is the chair? Who is in charge?

BOT: (Laughs a little) I don't know.

ACT-C: Play along a little. OK? Pretend—say you get to put one in charge.

BOT: OK. I'd put 'I'm just being realistic' in charge.

ACT-C: OK sounds great. (Whispered as if to keep other thoughts from hearing.) Realistic seems like the most sensible one in the mix—probably make a good chair—but don't tell the others I said so—wouldn't want to hurt their feelings.

Consulting from an ACT perspective needs to be consistent with the model both at the level of the content of the consultation and also at the level of process. In this dialogue, the ACT consultant has begun with an initial acknowledgement of the colleagues' value (being a useful therapist) and moved quickly to the obstacles to pursuit of that value. Note that the consultant in the above interaction does not respond literally to the content of the colleagues' thoughts. The consultant does not treat the thought that the colleague is "not a good therapist" as requiring refutation. Conventional responses in the above dialogue would likely involve some version of friendly refutation: "Now come on, you and I both know some of the tough cases you've seen." The well-meaning colleague might marshal examples of successful treatments, positive work evaluations, and praise from colleagues in order to counter the negative thoughts. Or, taking another tack, a conventional response might involve a sort of empathic joining: "Yeah, I guess we all feel that way some days." Although differing in form, both of these responses function to momentarily lessen the burden of negative thought and emotion.

The burned out therapist does not want to have these thoughts and has likely engaged in behaviors to reduce them including: trying not to think them, feeling relieved when they are not prominent, and feeling resigned when they are persistently present. He has also almost certainly already attempted to refute them. As above, although different in form, all of these behaviors are ways to reduce, eliminate, or at least to hunker down and weather the storm of negative cognition and emotion.

From an ACT perspective, we want to accomplish two things with respect to these negative thoughts: first, we want to make a functional analysis of the thoughts, and second, we want to begin to defuse them. Understanding the functional properties of the thoughts is accomplished by asking questions about what the thoughts "tell" our colleague to do. In this questioning, we begin to illuminate the functional similarity of the thoughts and also begin to accomplish our other goal: to help our colleague gain some psychological flexibility with respect to the thoughts. Defusion in this interaction, is facilitated by personifying the thought. The personification is enhanced by pretending not to want to hurt some of the thought's "feelings." The entire act of treating the thoughts as a sort of committee has a somewhat playful aspect. Helping our colleague to be playful with his thoughts is a different way of interacting than interacting with them as if the thoughts themselves were serious threats to his work and personal integrity. The act of examining these thoughts in this way also helps to bolster the ACT distinction between self-as-content and self-as-context. Although it is not stated explicitly in the dialogue, the distinction between thinker and thought has begun. All of these interactions are aimed at generating psychological flexibility in response to negative thoughts. Even though the thought is still highly believable, the consultant has sown the seeds of both defusion and the experience of self-as-context.

> ACT-C: I hear a sort of weariness in you though—like it is hard to go in each day and face it.
>
> BOT: Sure, but what else am I going to do. I have to go to work.
>
> ACT-C: It sounds like you have given up something that was important to you—like you've lost something—that sense that you might be able to sort of reach in and make a difference in someone's life. And, you have tried hard to fight off this weariness haven't you?
>
> BOT: Yes.
>
> ACT-C: What kinds of things have you tried?
>
> BOT: Well, I've tried to ignore those thoughts and just focus on my work. I've gone on holiday. I've been to a million seminars, poured over the journals—trying to find something new. I went to therapy myself for a while. We worked on focusing on the good that I was doing. And, it really is true. Some people really do better and are grateful.
>
> ACT-C: Sounds like that was helpful. What about the other things?
>
> BOT: Well, yes, it helped some, for a while. But really, I am just tired. Trying to keep a positive attitude just wears me out. I just don't feel like it!
>
> ACT-C: But all these things promised to work—to help you out with this weariness. And, they do help some.
>
> BOT: Yes, but it's just not enough. Nothing lasts. I end up as tired as before. There's just got to be more to it than this. Some days I can hardly get out of bed.

Here, the consultant touches on the colleagues' sense of hopelessness and then begins to explore the workability of the control agenda. The consultant does so without prejudice. If the ACT consultant concludes that things don't work, they risk denying experienced workability. There is certainly a modicum of workability in the colleague's agenda. It needs to be acknowledged. If the colleague's strategies to manage burnout were workable in a thoroughgoing way, however, the conversation would not be occurring. The ACT consultant persistently explores experienced workability, what workability works for, and seeks the experienced limits of that workability. It is these limits that have brought the colleague into the consultation.

ACT-C: Can I ask you something very personal? If there were something in your own experience of weariness that could help your clients, that could reconnect you to your work with them in a powerful way, would you be willing to let me ask about that? What if there is something right at the heart of that weariness that could be of extraordinary value to you? Would you be willing to go there?

BOT: Sure. I mean—I just don't know if I can keep this up.

ACT-C: OK. I want to start by asking an odd question. Imagine I had a magic button right here. Press it and you go to work, and, as now, you are reasonably effective, you keep your job, but you become sort of immune to your clients—remember this is magic. So, with this new immunity, you sit in there and listen to the same old stories, but you feel fine—like the radio playing in the background. If they do incredibly poorly, you are unaffected. But it is also the case that if they do incredibly well, you experience the same indifference. It just doesn't matter to you, and, this is important, *it doesn't matter that it doesn't matter*. You don't care about your clients, and you don't care that you don't care. Would you push the button?

BOT: Well no! They need someone who cares about them.

ACT-C: Yes, but remember push the button, and that fact doesn't bother you anymore. And, let me raise the ante: imagine that you can also completely fool them. You look exactly like someone who cares. They will never know how little you care about them.

BOT: No! I don't want to trick them, I want to help them!

ACT-C: OK. More magic: I want you to imagine a world in which there is a buffet. You step over to the buffet. You can have anything you want. In the first tray you have "lousy therapist," in the second, "mediocre therapist," in the third, "OK therapist," in the fourth, "good therapist," and, in the fifth pan they are serving "extraordinary, effective therapist." If you could chose any one of them, which would you chose. Remember, you chose it and it is yours—instantly.

BOT: Well, would chose the last one, of course, but I can't just choose it. It's not possible.

ACT-C: Sure, but I'm not asking about possible right now. We can come back to that. Right now I am just trying to get what you want. If I could just hold it out and offer it, would you want it? When you were being trained, was that what you dreamed of…when you let yourself dream?

BOT: Yes. I mean sure.

ACT-C: OK, let me just check in a little further. You know the weariness you talked to me about before.

BOT: Sure.

ACT-C: Just a little more magic: Imagine that I can offer you two choices. If you chose from this hand, the weariness you feel, the sadness, the hopelessness, all goes away. Poof! Never again, for the rest of your life, do you feel it. But there is a cost. That indifference we talked about before, with clients, you feel that for everyone on the planet. Your wife, kids, clients, everyone. If your kids come to you troubled….nothing, you haven't the slightest sense of what they are feeling, *and,* as before, it doesn't bother you a bit that you don't. In my other hand, I have another choice. Over here, you feel that pain, sadness, weariness, as many days a year as you feel it now, forever, but somehow, even feeling all that, you find that you can truly feel the clients you serve. When they speak to you, you can truly hear them. And your children, when they come to you and say, 'Dad, sometimes I feel so unsure of myself. I'm afraid that I will never be able to do anything right.' When they come and say that, you can hear them and feel their pain, in that moment—and they can tell that they have been understood. But don't forget, with this choice, you bring all of your own pain along.

BOT: I don't want the pain.

ACT-C: (quiet) I know. But, if that were the choice? If it were, what would you choose?

BOT: I would choose the pain. If it meant I could really be there for my clients, and especially for my wife and kids.

ACT-C: I got it. I hear you.

In this segment, the main work component is the clarification of the colleagues' values and making those values psychologically present in the consultation. We will rely on those values to orient and dignify the consultation. Although professing indifference, the therapist' valuing of his clients and others in his life is clarified in this series of choices. No effort is made to point out the logical inconsistency of the BOT's professed indifference in the face of his clear caring for his clients that is expressed by his willingness to choose pain in their service.

Although the focus is on values, there are several other ACT components at work in this interaction. The BOT experiences his negative emotions and thoughts as literally dangerous to his efficacy and to his integrity. The thought that he does not care for his clients, for example, is regarded as literally true. Rather than argue with the content, the ATC-C gets the colleague engaged with these negative thoughts and feelings in a different way. The consultant sets the occasion for the BOT to act with integrity in the face of these thoughts and feelings. The very act of choosing to have negative thoughts and feelings fosters the distinction between thought and thinker, felt and feeler—and therefore facilitates defusion and the BOT's sense of self-as-context.

These are different interactions with negative cognition and emotion than are usual for this individual's typical attempts to suppress and avoid. Broadening of repertoire is the hallmark of defusion. In this way, values and defusion are inextricably linked in ACT interventions and consultations. As the BOT interacts in a rich and articulated way with previously avoided material the domination of that material lessens.

> ACT-C: Now I want to ask about the impossible part. Tell me why you can't have the thing you value. What is between you and 'being an extraordinary and engaged therapist?' Imagine we are writing a novel about someone just like you. What is the story? Imagine the story starts like this: "He wanted to be an extraordinary therapist, but…." I'll write the "buts" under the heading of "The Story."

Together, the ACT-C and BOT fill out the following table including the story, what the story equals, and, what strategies he has tried in order to solve the problem.

The Story	Equals	Strategies
I just don't feel the compassion I once felt for clients	= get more compassion	1. conceal how I actually feel 2. think about how to acquire compassion 3. think about changing jobs
Maybe I'm just tired of doing rehab	= get more enthusiasm	1. conceal how I actually feel 2. think hard about changing jobs 3. try to talk myself into excitement
I feel burned out	= get more energy/conserve energy	1. take time off 2. work at low level
I'm not sure if I was meant to be a therapist	= get more clarity about my career	1. think hard about career choice
Maybe I am just not that good	= improve myself	1. take classes 2. read technical material 3. go to workshops
What I wanted wasn't realistic	= be satisfied with the way things "really are"	1. talk myself into being satisfied
I'm stuck, just stuck	= find a way to get unstuck	1. think hard about a way out of the trap

ACT-C: You have years of experience with these solutions and you have an education about how to solve problems. Let's look at your experience of how they have served you. Imagine your valued direction is true north on a compass. We'll look at each one of these strategies and see if, in your experience, they have moved you north.

Equals	Strategies	Short term	Long term
= get more compassion	1. conceal how I actually feel 2. think about how to acquire compassion 3. think about changing jobs	1. yes, I think I can hide my lack of compassion most days 2. no change 3. it feels appealing sometimes, but not for long	1. no, feel even more disconnected, phony, mechanical 2. no change 3. no change
= get more enthusiasm	1. conceal how I actually feel 2. think hard about changing jobs 3. try to talk myself into excitement	1. I think I can look enthusiastic some days 2. no change 3. no change	1. no, feel even more disconnected, phony 2. no change 3. no change
= get more energy/conserve energy	1. take time off 2. work at low level	1. felt great at the moment 2. doesn't really help	1. no 2. no, I end up feeling more and more burned out
= get more clarity about my career	1. think hard about career choice	1. feels appealing for a while, but doesn't last	1. no, the longer I think, the less clear I feel
= improve myself	1. take classes 2. read technical material 3. go to workshops	1. not really, hard to stay focused 2. boring 3. get excited for a while, but it fades	1. no change 2. no change 3. no change over the long run
= be satisfied with the way things "really are"	1. talk myself into being satisfied	1. not really	1. no, just a lot of energy wasted arguing with myself
= find a way to get unstuck	1. think hard about a way out of the trap	1. not really	1. lots of energy, and nothing changes

ACT-C: What is the workability of these strategies? Have you gotten closer or farther away from your value as a therapist?

BOT: Obviously, farther away. But that's what I said in the beginning, I am more realistic today.

ACT-C: And when you say you have given up, let's look at that thought. Does that thought move you towards your values, or away from them?

BOT: Further away. Maybe I should change jobs.

ACT-C: And the thought that you should change professions, where does that lead you?

BOT: I feel like a failure.

ACT-C: And where does 'I feel like a failure' take you? Does it feel vital? Does it feel like it moves you towards what you value?

BOT: No. It's the same old thing. It goes nowhere.

ACT-C: So when you are in therapy, and this lethargy, this self-doubt, this disconnection comes over you, what do you actually do?

BOT: Well, we have pretty defined procedures. I do the steps of the functional analysis. I follow along with the protocol. As long as I stick to the protocol, I can keep anything from leaking out....most days. But, it is so tiring. The whole time I am just waiting for the day to end.

ACT-C: Let me ask you this: have you noticed this spilling over outside work?

BOT: Yes, I feel it at home too. I just keep my head down. Bury myself in a book or television. But, I just don't know how to get what I want.

ACT-C: Ok, so this is where you find yourself. If you could pick, like at the buffet I mentioned, where would you choose to go?

BOT: I want to be compassionate and close. I want to be useful.

ACT-C: The question is, when you look at your experience, of how have these strategies functioned for you, have they moved you closer to your clients, you family? And, if they haven't, are you willing to give them up?

BOT: No, I am not. I don't have any other alternatives. If I don't have them, I would really be sunk, I would have nothing to offer.

ACT-C: Do you recognize this "stuck" place you are in right now from the "stuckness" of your clients? They want to get rid of their pain first before going on with their lives in the same way you want to get rid of the feelings of lethargy before you go on. Your clients are as sure they are right about these solutions as you are about yours. And yet, neither of you are moving forward towards the places you want to go. Do you recognize that "stuckness?"

BOT: Yea, I guess I do. But I don't want to see it. Those strategies have worked at times. They are not completely worthless. They are reasonable solutions.

ACT-C. Sure, sometimes purposeful, planful approaches work fine. Even in the areas we have talked about, they can have temporary effects. Like when you told me about taking time off. Not that there is anything wrong with taking time off, but what was the long-term effect? Look to your clients too. Some of them have been off work for years. Do the ones who have been off work the longest look happiest? Or, the least stressed?

BOT: No. Not really. But what alternative do I have—should I just give up?

ACT-C: And that—giving up—is that familiar? Haven't you already tried that too?

BOT: Yes—very familiar. But what am I supposed to do?

ACT-C: What would happen if you let go of this struggle with how you feel?

BOT: It would just bury me. I mean, I would become useless? I would fall apart. Who would want a therapist or a dad or a friend who is incompetent?

The above exchange is an example of relentless appeal to process. The content of thoughts is not engaged. Instead, each thought is put to the functional acid test: does this move you in the direction of a vital, fulfilling life? Ignoring content and focusing on process alters the context of usual social discourse. The ordinary response to "I feel like a failure" would be to argue against it. To the extent that we alter this altogether ordinary and well-meaning response, we defuse the life restricting functions of such thoughts. In this segment, the ACT-C also focuses on the aspects of creative hopelessness and the agenda of control. In the next segment, the ACT-C takes the colleague into a very specific professional example in order to coach an alternative to the agenda of control.

ACT-C: Ok, I want you to think about a client about whom who you are most worried.

BOT: OK. I have one in mind—a woman I have been treating—terrible situation.

ACT-C: So tell me—if things go the way of your worst fears, what happens. Just take a moment and let those worst fears show up. (long pause) What happens?

BOT: (quiet) She dies. I worry that she won't be able to hang on.

ACT-C: I would like to do a little exercise with you. I will ask you to imagine a few things and will ask a few questions. Please don't open your eyes or stop the exercise. Just answer briefly as you can. Close your eyes for a few minutes and imagine that you are walking in to your therapy room to see this woman. On this particular imagined day, you have set aside your agenda, your manual, and your protocol. Let yourself picture the day, the room, her face before you.

BOT: It is very scary. What would I do without an agenda? Behavior therapists always have a clipboard and a planned agenda.

ACT-C. On this day you don't. You walk into that room with no idea what will happen. You have no diagnosis, and no agenda. How does that feel?

BOT: Scary! Very scary! Having a clipboard and an agenda makes me feel more secure, more professional. I would feel naked not having anything with me.

ACT-C: Notice your own struggle….how much you want to have a plan. And, now, just for a moment, see if you can let go of that struggle and just allow yourself to feel what you feel. Take a moment and as if you had a list before you, I want you to notice some things. Let each thing you notice appear on the list, and when it is there on the list imagine that you place a check beside it, and then go on to notice the next thing. First, notice your body, how it feels, take a moment and let all of the sensations you notice in your body appear on the list, one at a time, and just check each off as you notice it. (long pause) Now notice the different emotions you are experiencing in the same way. Let them show up on the list and check them off. (long pause) And, now, notice and thoughts or memories, take your time, see if you can catch and release each one. (long pause) Now, I want you to see if you can let go of any attachment to the sensations, emotions, thoughts, memories. If you notice yourself being very drawn to one, go ahead and pick it up, note it on you list, and gently, as soon as you can….release it. (long pause) Now I want you to come back to the face of your client. Picture yourself with her again in the room. All you are doing is sitting, face to face with another human being and showing up for that person in front of you. I want you to imagine just looking into her eyes. See if you can see the person behind those eyes. See if you can let go of her "problem" for a just a minute and see the person there. Listen to her voice, feel her struggle and disappointments. Allow yourself to feel her pain and struggle as she tries to tell you why she is there.

BOT. Yes, that feels very different but scary. I can feel her pain and suffering. But then what? How am I supposed to help her if I don't have an agenda?

ACT-C: For just a moment, I want you to let go of the problem solving agenda. You can pick it up again in a moment, but for right now, see if you can just let yourself hear her, let yourself see her. And, now, I want you to gently come back into this room, with me, and open your eyes. What do you feel?

BOT: I feel compassion for her.

ACT-C. And in this moment—this very moment, do you feel that lethargy, or do you feel vitality…life?

BOT: Life.

ACT-C. And in this moment—this very moment, do you feel that stuckness—that sense of being completely bound, or does it feel as though you have just a bit more room to live your life? Do you feel more burdened or less?

BOT: More free, a little lighter.

ACT-C: I want to stop a second here and notice what just happened. You began by saying that you no longer felt compassion for your clients, that you felt no motivation. You listed all of the things that you did to try to change these thoughts and feelings–time off, taking course, considering changing jobs, trying to give yourself a pep talk. But notice what just happened here. You experienced a little bit of freedom–a little bit of life. No new knowledge, no figuring anything out! Let's look at what we did: I started by asking you what you cared about. I asked you about obstacles. Then we took a few minutes letting go of the struggle. And finally, I asked you, in the exercise, to make psychological contact with the pain of your most difficult, your most frightening client. Weird, huh? We went into the problem, moved around, and found more psychological space for you to reconnect with your vocation. When you allow yourself to feel this compassion, are you nearer or further away from the therapist you want to be?

BOT: Closer. I think my client could feel my empathy for her.

In this segment of the consultation, the experiential exercise is used as a venue to coach foster mindfulness and acceptance with respect to disturbing thoughts. This defusion work is carried out in the context of the colleague's most difficult client, which makes more likely the difficult material, and in the context of the colleague's value. Following the exercise, the therapist capitalizes on the immediate experience to do discrimination training for aspects of experience that distinguish values-consistent acceptance as opposed to values-inconsistent avoidance.

BOT: But how does that help the problem? She still has the same problem she came in with. How does my feeling compassion help? I'm a behavior therapist. You are starting to sound like a psychodynamic therapist. What is this?

ACT-C: What if what we are talking about right now, about connecting and feeling compassion for other human beings doesn't belong to any therapy school? What if this ability to connect to other human beings is something we all have regardless of education or background. What if this connection is the basis of the therapeutic alliance?

BOT: As a behavior therapist, I was taught to have an agenda all prepared before I walked in the room. I was taught to structure all the information into a behavior analysis of the problem and then to look for the latest research about how to treat that diagnosis.

ACT-C: I'm not saying that there is anything wrong with treatment protocols or manuals. I am just saying that the first step is to ally with the client. How does it feel to you when you are around someone who always knows the answers—someone who immediately gives advice whenever any problem comes up?

BOT: I don't like them much. I guess sometimes I doubt that they are so smart. Or, even when I do think they are smart, I don't want to be around them. It just reminds me of my own problems.

ACT-C: How safe does it feel to talk to them?

BOT: Not safe at all. I stay quiet and I stay *away* if I can.

ACT-C: And when you are in therapy? How safe are you—for your clients? Who are you? Are you the one who knows all the answers?

BOT: I guess I hide behind those protocols. I wouldn't want the client to see my vulnerability.

ACT-C: Why not? What would be dangerous about showing yourself?

BOT: They would probably complain about me. They want me to be big and strong. I am supposed to be helping them.

ACT-C. They might, and that is a risk. But by putting on a show that you are big and strong in order to hide those feelings, what has that resulted in?

BOT: That I don't have the contact I want anyway. They might leave me because we have no closeness anymore. And if they do stay, I still feel disconnected.

ACT-C. It sounds like you are taking risks either way. So which way do you choose? Do you want to keep hiding and playing big to avoid those feelings of weakness or do you want to allow yourself to feel vulnerable and show that vulnerability and in so doing give yourself a chance to give that compassion that you prize?

BOT: But what then? What about helping them with their problems?

ACT-C: It depends what you think the problem is. Is your job to reduce their feelings of pain, anxiety, and depression or is your job to help them get on with their lives?

BOT. Both, first I have to help them manage those all of that negativity and then I help them get on with their lives. I use cognitive techniques to reframe the dysfunctional thoughts and make them less credible and then I go on to using exposure to reduce anxiety and pain. Then I give homework assignments so that the client can apply exposure in their everyday lives.

ACT-C. How does that agenda work usually?

BOT: It's tiring—hard to get them to do the work—especially homework. The exposure part is also aversive to me and to the client. Usually I work with the physical therapist and the occupational therapists. We ask the client what causes them pain. They show us how a certain movement of activity causes pain. Then we just simulate it. If they say, for example that making a bed or lifting a box elicits pain than we would simulate that situation and ask them to do that movement or activity.

ACT-C: How do you get them to do that when they say it causes them pain?

BOT: We persuade them. We tell them that we have experience with this. We tell them about our evaluations. We say that if they do this they will get better by the end of this program. It is hard. Most of the exposure gets done when we stand over them.

ACT-C: How does the interaction feel when you are doing that exposure work?

BOT: Well, it doesn't feel like you are their friend. They do it because they have to. It's crazy. I am trying to help them, but sometimes it feels more like I am policing them.

ACT-C: And, how does it feel when someone is standing over you watching you to make sure you do a difficult job? How does it feel when your supervisor comes and looks over your files?

BOT: Well, like I am being policed—punitive.

ACT-C: What do we know about the effects of punishment?

BOT: That the behavior can be eliminated temporarily and the side effects for the person receiving the punishment are fear and negative feelings towards the person who is giving the punishment. Are you suggesting that we are punishing our clients by using exposure?

ACT-C: I am saying that exposure for its own sake with no context *could be* perceived by the person it is being done as punishment. I don't think we intend to, but I do think that sometimes we don't spend as much time as we might connecting with the "why" of exposure.

BOT: There is a context. We tell the client that most everyone who goes through exposure gets better.

ACT-C: That is your context not the client's. Where is the client's context for exposure? Why would they be motivated to undergo a painful procedure?

BOT: Because I tell them the statistics of how many people get better.

ACT-C: Imagine that you are the client and you know from your own experience that doing certain activities has caused you terrible pain in the past, and a therapist is telling you that you need to do just those activities that you know will hurt. You think this sounds crazy but the therapist is trying to persuade you by telling you a bunch of statistics about the average patient and significances, which means nothing to you at all. You also know from the insurance company that you have to comply with the program or loose you disability payments. What do you do?

BOT: I would do what I had to do to keep my disability payment but no more.

ACT-C. How would you, as the client, do with homework assignments?

BOT: I would not do them and make up excuses.

ACT-C: How about the sessions where you argue with the therapist about your thought patterns?

BOT: I wouldn't mind arguing, but I wouldn't change my mind. Nobody likes being told how to think.

ACT-C. That's probably right, nobody likes to be told what to do at all? What if there is another way to come at that hard work?

BOT. How else could exposure be done?

ACT-C: In exactly the way you and I just worked with your feelings of weariness and failure. What if the psychological pain you experience, that seems to be *forcing* you out of work is like the physical pain experienced by your clients? What was your reason for exposing yourself and showing me your vulnerabilities? Did you feel forced into anything.

BOT: No. I did it because I want to be a better therapist. Because I miss that connection I used to have with my work and my clients.

ACT-C: Why should clients expose themselves to pain? Partly the answer to this depends on what you think exposure is for. Do you think exposure is to reduce pain or is it to reduce disability? As to the pain part, well you and I both know that sometimes pain goes and sometimes it doesn't. We can't make big promises about pain going away. It does when it does. But, what if we think about exposure as being about reducing disability, or better still, about increasing life? Og Lindsley used to tell people not to pick a behavioral target that a dead person could do better. So, if our goal is to reduce distress, we are giving our clients a target that a dead person could accomplish. The dead feel no pain. But, the dead can't be good fathers, husbands, *therapists.*

BOT: Ok, I get what you're saying. My client and I are in the same boat. So, let me run through this process again. Step 1 is establishing the therapeutic alliance. I think I understand what you mean there. I need to just connect and allow myself to feel compassion for the client. But how do I get the clients context?

ACT-C. In exactly the same way we looked at yours—but more broadly. You ask the client two important questions: What do you want and what are you afraid of? What we did was in the domain of work, but we could have as easily done the same thing in other areas of your life where you feel constricted—cut off. You said yourself that you feel the way some of the malaise at work spills over into other areas of living. Isn't it the same for our pain patients? It starts by interfering with work, but does it stop there? You can use values interventions in the same way we just did to establish the client's context.

BOT: Ok, so step one is getting connected, step two is establishing the context of what the clients wants, step three is finding out what the client is afraid of and what is next.

ACT-C: Exposure is still the key element in therapy. Exposure is one of our most powerful tools. The difference here, however, is that exposure will be baked in the client's context–in the client's values. More strangeness still, eh: client-centered behavior therapy! The motivation for exposure to painful feelings would be that the client will be moving in a valued direction, not doing what you tell them is good for them.

BOT. How would I do exposure? What about those homework exercises?

ACT-C: Once you have helped the client to establish their valued directions, the obstacles and helped to defuse the stories, and accept negative feelings, they often start moving on their own. If you do create homework exercises with them, you create exercises that move them towards the life they want. You can also use exposure exercises like I did with you. Once you know what they are afraid of, you can include these negative experiences in guided imagery and help them to "feel" and be willing to accept negative private events–always in the service of the life they want. Like when you were willing to feel uncertain if it helped make you a better therapist. Notice when we did that exercise, I asked you to become mindful of all of those difficult thoughts and feelings, then I coached letting go of the struggle, and then we came back to the thing you value–being there for your clients.

BOT: Ok so guided imagery in exposure. How do I do diffusion exercises? What does that mean?

ACT-C: Diffusion or deliteralization aims at seeing thoughts as what they are and not what they say they are. The different exercises attempt to expand attention to thinking and experiencing as an ongoing behavioral process. Many of the exercises use mindfulness or role-play to create some space in between the person and the thoughts and feelings. You can have thoughts and feelings without being these thoughts and feelings. Many of the verbal rules clients use lead them away from where they want to be going. The functional analysis you do will be based on going forward and building towards valued directions. Obstacles are taken up as they try to block the road.

BOT. That sounds much more fun that listening to problems all the time. What about the homework assignments?

ACT-C: Put yourself in that situation. If you have identified your valued direction and you recognize the thoughts and feelings that will try and stop you and you have made a commitment to put your feet towards your valued intentions, what would you do? If I were to ask you this, you have identified compassion as a valued direction in your meetings with clients. What will you do in your next meeting with your client?

BOT: I will slow down and create that space and allow myself to feel that compassion for myself and for the client.

ACT-C: How would it have affected you if I had given you a homework assignment before you have thought that action through?

BOT: I would probably have thought that you knew better how I should do this. Maybe I would have resented that you told me what to do.

ACT-C: Now, if we were to talk in terms of homework, I might give you suggestions about how to go about that. For example, remember that really difficult client you spoke of? I might suggest that you spend the first few minutes of your next session with her doing an eyes-closed, mindfulness exercise with her. Just spend the first few minutes directing her to look back over the week and notice, then release the different difficult things she has experienced, then spend a few minutes quiet—eyes still closed—focusing on the in and outflow of breath. Do the exercise with her. Then ask her to open her eyes, you open yours, and just sit for a moment quiet and see if you can see the person behind those eyes that is working so hard to be OK, or to have a good excuse for not being OK.....just like you. This little bit of homework is organic. It grows naturally from what you want.

BOT: I see what you mean. The client is motivated by the natural positive reinforcement that is in that situation rather than doing it for me as a homework exercise.

ACT-C: Try and see.

The order of ACT interventions, including consultation and training, is often do-then-say. In this relatively didactic component of the consultation, the ACT-C points back to the colleague's experience in the consultation, and maps that experience onto the colleague's professional activity. ACT principles are scalable. The principles that apply in consultation also apply in therapy. This has several advantages. The BOT in this consultation the colleague's sources of difficulty in his work are addressed directly with standard ACT components as they apply to the colleagues work. In addition, the colleague is given a new way of working with clients. Of course, doing ACT would require additional training. However, the interaction sets the stage for both acceptance and change—acceptance of challenging thoughts and emotions that are part and parcel of working with difficult clients and change in the form of modifications to the therapy provided.

Summary of the Dialogue

Working with clients who are stuck is a challenge to all therapists. Shutting down our compassion and empathy will seriously restrict our ability to help them. Spending our energy trying to look competent in order to disguise our vulnerability is likely to be a great strain. We will get tired and feel stressed. From an ACT perspective problems of stress and burn-out are compounded by experiential avoidance. This is not to say that workload is irrelevant, but the relationship between workload and burn-out is not simple. The model suggests that whatever stresses occur may be compounded depending upon our relationship with those stressors. At least in some instances, our trouble may not be so much the result of feeling compassion for our client's suffering, but because we are trying to protect ourselves from feeling it. Applying ACT principles to ourselves, and our work, can be a way to identify and rectify therapist burn-out.

Integrating ACT into Treatment Teams

It is possible to infuse ACT sensibilities into supervision teams and treatment teams. In some instances, we may have buy-in from the group and have permission to organize the work of the treatment team with a sensitivity to these issues. Although it is beyond the scope of this volume, a few suggestions can be made.

Participation and Choice

First and foremost, experiential acceptance and willingness cannot be forced. Taking an accepting posture towards the psychological challenges that occur in the treatment of refractory clients needs to be chosen by each of the team members. *And*, even when it has been chosen, it needs to be re-chosen again and again. In order to organize such a group, we have to have a level of acceptance that we and others in the group will do a better and worse job depending on the day. Our experience in therapy, and in supervision, suggests a degree of humility is in order. Engaging in such activity is always by invitation. What we can create is an environment that invites and fosters experiential openness and psychological flexibility. We do this by openly discussing and supporting one another in discussing the "hard facts" of our work. We do so because sometimes the "hard facts" overwhelm the *other facts*. Sometimes the pain causes us to forget the humanity of the individuals before us, their willingness to bear suffering for a purpose; the humanity of our colleagues as they sit with those who are in pain, who continue on, committed, in the face of a "mindfield" of objective and subjective difficulty.

Building a Mission

A commitment to building an environment that supports psychological flexibility means attending to the factors that inhibit flexibility. Some of these factors will be endemic in the work we do. Aversive events generate inflexibility. Our clients come to us in pain. It is painful to watch people be in pain. It is painful to coach people to do things that, at least initially, increase pain. And, finally, it is painful to watch someone not do what will need doing in order for them to move ahead in their life. What makes this pain worthwhile? In the previous section, we suggested openly discussing, coaching and fostering willingness. We do this in the context of values.

Often mission statements are things that upper administration wants to see on paper. Often, for the people whose mission is described, the statements have little personal relevance, or at least, the relevance is abstract. This need not be the case.

The development of a mission statement that the people on the team can personally endorse provides a guiding star for the workgroup. Just as in sailing, we need a point that is both high and constant. Ideally, a mission statement should address both content and process. Mission statements often address issues of content: "This hospital is dedicated to serving...." Less frequently, mission statements address the processes by which the content mission will accomplished. Our experience suggests that explicitly stating, and reiterating, our commitment to an open process is worthwhile.

A Few Group Process Issues

Appreciation. Surrounded by so many problems, it is easy to slip into the problem solving mode. Problem solving is great. However, not everything is a problem to be solved. Problems quite naturally draw our attention and restrict our capacity to appreciate what else is present. We can explicitly bring into the culture of the workgroup. When a colleague is struggling to help a very difficult client, we can pause a moment and acknowledge the dignity of the care that is offered. Appreciation ought to be genuine. Just as with mission statements, we do not want appreciation to be hollow and formal. Very often acts of heartfelt appreciation create a context for others to pause and appreciate. It is difficult to put too much appreciation in any environment. Try it at home. Try it the next time you are at the grocery store. Try it with your spouse or children. Just stop a minute. Look for something you can appreciate—even a very simple thing, like a nice smile. When you have found it and felt it—say it out loud. Watch the effect it has. Appreciation does not make problems go away. It just helps us to hold the problems in context.

Complaining. The opposite ought to be explicitly avoided. Complaining, especially about co-workers, can be very toxic. Don't participate in it. Walk away from it when you see it. Complaints about co-workers tend to harden their position. Whatever is complained about must be defended. Worse still, it creates subgroups and loyalties within the subgroups that masquerade as benevolent, but subvert the efforts of the team as a whole. We need to look carefully at the function of evaluation. If we are in a position to hire and fire, evaluation might be a difficult, but necessary, task. However, more typically our complaining does nothing except poison the interpersonal waters from which we must then drink. If there is not a direct action implied by the evaluation, consider setting evaluation aside. This does not mean changing a negative evaluation to a positive evaluation. It also does not mean that we turn off evaluation—like a light switch. The process is more like a meditation in which the task is to let go of unproductive evaluation when we find ourselves engaged in it and come back to the task—perhaps remembering that on our worst days, we, like them, find ourselves several miles from perfect. Again, this fostering of appreciation and stepping away from complaining is everyone's job—always shared, never divided. In ACT parlance, we are always response-able, if we are willing. This matter can be described directly in the mission of the group.

Periodic Recommitment to and Reconnecting with the Mission

Being part of a group with a mission means losing track of the mission. The day-to-day troubles come to dominate our activity. Ironically, regular meetings that let go of day-to-day problems in order to reconnect and recommit to the mission can sometimes set a context where day-to-day problems can be usefully engaged. This sort of activity can sometimes appear a waste of precious hours. However, if we examine our daily lives, we often find that raw hours is not the deciding factor. Some hours are far more productive than others. Making contact with the meaning of our work and with the meaning of our work to our fellows can set a context for highly productive activity.

Bringing Process into the Meetings

There are both experiential and technical aspects of doing ACT that can be explored experientially and didactically in team meetings. Taking time out at the beginning of a meeting for an experiential and/or mindfulness exercises can both help us to be more present in the meeting that follows, can help us to become more fluent in these techniques, and finally can set the stage for discussions of important technical and stylistic aspects involved in using these procedures. Values and commitment exercises, for example, in the context of the meeting on group mission described in the previous section can serve several functions. As with mindfulness and other experiential exercises, these exercises can set the stage for discussion of both the experience of doing the exercise as well as with technical aspects of executing the exercise. Watching ourselves and others do this task allows us to become familiar with an exercise we will ask clients to do. In addition, as we watch our colleagues stand up and make commitments, it humanizes them, and draws us together as a working group.

Conclusion

Even when we do not have *carte blanche* to organize a workgroup around these principles, there are ways that aspects of these processes can be introduced piecemeal. For example, because the use of mindfulness in the treatment of chronic pain has gained some prominence in recent years the introduction of mindfulness type exercises might be acceptable.

Assignment

Consider a client you are working with about whom you are most worried. Spend a few minutes, eyes closed. Allow yourself to settle and become mindful. Allow yourself to imagine that your worst fear for this client has happened. Imagine that you are completely unable to help them and that your worst fears come true.

Following this exercise, spend a few minutes answering the following questions:

1) When you are seeing your most difficult clients, what are your typical reactions to their difficult thoughts and feelings?

2) What difficult thoughts and emotions do you experience?

3) What is your relationship with your own difficult thoughts and feelings?

4) In what ways are your interactions with difficult psychological material consistent or inconsistent with an ACT model?

5) Do these ways of interacting with your client and your own difficult psychological material facilitate movement in a vital direction?

Chapter 10

A Brief ACT Intervention for Clients with Longstanding Stress and Pain Symptoms

The aim of this chapter is to present an example of an actual ACT pain protocol. While the treatment protocol presented here is designed to be implemented in a very brief format, there are other ACT protocols that allow for longer-term treatment strategies. A well-developed example is McCracken et al. (in press). They describe an ACT-based intervention strategy that unfolds in multiple sessions over a period of three-to-four weeks, and is designed to help patients with disabling chronic pain regain some of their day-to-day functioning. The results of the study were generally quite positive: subjects showed significant improvement the areas of social, physical and emotional functioning, and did not require a concomitant reduction of pain symptoms to do so. We will describe this protocol and its results in a bit more detail at the end of this chapter.

Not all therapists have the luxury of a four-week multi-disciplinary course of treatment, however. Fortunately, ACT-based strategies lend themselves well to very brief interventions protocols, and they have been shown to be effective even with severe clients in this format (e.g., see Bach & Hayes, 2002). This does not necessarily mean that a short ACT intervention is likely to be as effective as a more extensive one, but rather that short interventions can be quite useful.

What follows is a description of a research protocol used for the treatment of individuals with longstanding pain and stress symptoms, and who were also on long-term disability leave from work (Dahl et al., 2004). The individual elements of this protocol have already been fairly extensively described in this volume, but this chapter will show how they can be sequenced in a coherent whole. We will be walking through them more in outline form, but with some clinical comments along the way.

Part of the purpose in doing so is to show that even relatively focused ACT interventions can have a major impact on human functioning, and to give the reader the sense that implementing ACT is indeed within the realm of the possible. The issues addressed in an ACT model are profound – they are central to human functioning. So far the data suggests that by raising these issues properly, large changes can occur even in a fairly short time, with fairly limited intervention. The present protocol is not complicated, and it is not extensive. And yet our data suggests that it makes a big difference.

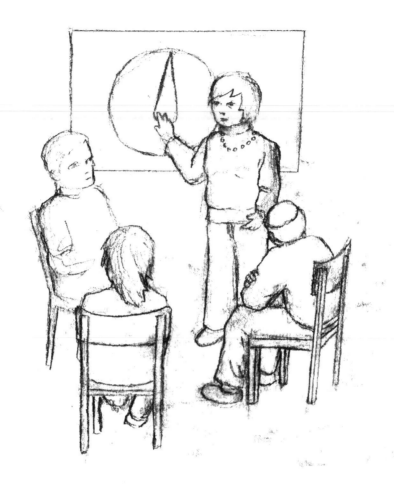

ACT Treatment of Chronic Pain:
A Four-Session Mixed Individual and Group Protocol

The clients chosen for this particular program were those who reported debilitating pain, stress, and fatigue symptoms which prevented them from working, or functioning generally in typical daily activities. These individuals had participated in one or more rehabilitation programs but failed to recover. All of them had been on disability leave from work for between one and two years, and all of them were taking a variety of medication for pain, anxiety, depression, and sleep. Quality of life was greatly reduced for all the participants as a result of their struggle with chronic pain.

The typical characteristics of the individuals in this treatment group were as follows:

Behavior: Avoidance of activities, movements, and places associated with pain. This usually includes: work, work like activities, and work like movements.

Thoughts: Focus on short-term symptom alleviation, and verbal rules with the theme that pain and stress preclude normal living activities.

Physiological reaction: heightened sensitivity to pain and stress signals.

The aim of this four-session protocol was to build a broader and more flexible behavioral repertoire around the "fixed" reactions to the symptoms of pain and stress, and to increase life quality. The design of the treatment protocol was: Baseline measurements taken in one individual session, followed by two group sessions, and concluding with one final individual session.

Here is an outline of the treatment:

Session One: Individual
1. The therapist validates suffering and personal loss of life quality as indicated in the VLQ. A life compass is created based on the VLQ, including client intentions.
2. Demonstrate, via functional analysis, the barriers to acting consistently with intentions.
3. Do a functional analysis showing the futility of attempts to control stress and pain. Have clients make a commitment in lining up feet with intentions.

Session Two: Group (8 – 10 clients; 3 hours)
1. Discuss what happened when the client attempted to move feet in valued directions.
2. Introduce the concept of "stories" and the functional analysis of language.
3. Introduce the concept of acceptance of negative feelings, and practice it in the form of a mindfulness exercise.
3. Identify core fears or unpleasant feelings underlying the barriers to putting feet and intention in alignment, and practice exposure to these fears.
4. Verbalize commitments to aligning feet and intentions.

Session Three: Group (8 – 10 clients; 3 hours)
1. The funeral exercise.
2. Clients wrote "stories" (reasons for not acting in consistency with values) down. This was followed by a card game, in which cards were first avoided and then accepted.
3. Exposure using mindfulness exercise is applied to the negative feelings involved that week in attempting to put feet in line with intentions.
4. Commitment to acting in line with intentions is reiterated, and common barriers are identified and addressed.

Session Four: Individual
1. The individual clients present their life compasses, functional analyses of their "stories" and other relevant obstacles to behaviour change.
2. Independent presentation of strategies of acceptance and exposure.
3. Clients make a commitment to aligning activities with intentions as identified in compass.

Each session included an emphasis on these key components: values, exposure, cognitive defusion, and empowerment. Here is a more detailed analysis of how each component plays out in a session-by-session breakdown.

Session 1: Individual Session

1. Validation of suffering and consequential loss of life quality (approximately 5 minutes)
Start session with *validation of suffering*, considering the losses which the person has indicated in the questionnaire: (VLQ). Pose the question: How have these problems (symptoms) influenced your life, and what kind of losses have you experienced because them?

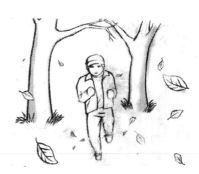

2. Values
Go to a white board with the client or use a blank piece of paper.
Importance
Draw ten circles, the client in the middle (ideally a picture is used), and label the circles as specific life dimensions (see Chapter 6). Ask the client to help rate the importance (0-10) of each life dimension *generally* (not only at the present time). These domains should not be rated relative to each other. Ask client to put their rating in a small box next to each circle.

Note: If the values of importance for each of these life dimensions are not all rated ten or close to it, you should note this. If any of the dimensions are very low you must be clear that you are not asking them to rate their present situation or how they feel "right now," but rather the category's general importance in their lives. If they still rate the dimension low, you need to further ask them why they put a lower rating on that particular dimension. It could be a choice or it could be a measure of a long-term adaptation ("I will rate it low because I can never do anything about it anyway") which is not healthy and needs to be looked into further.
Intentions
Ask the client to write a few words about each dimension describing how he/she would most like the dimension to be represented in their lives. No barriers should be accepted here, only a concrete picture of how what this dimension would look like under ideal circumstances. An example of this could be as follows: The client has said that having a social network is valued at 10. The concrete intention could be that "I meet friends regularly, have fun, and feel a sense of community and

belonging with them." These intentions do not need to be practically reachable. They can be "feelings" that the client is striving for such as "being present and mindful when spending time with my children." The intentions need to be identifiable and recognizable to the client. Label this drawing as the client's Life Compass.

Consistency

Ask the client to think about his/her activities in the past week, and ask how closely these activities coincided with the intention of each life dimension. In other words, in what direction did your feet go? Did your feet follow your intentions or did they go somewhere else? Ask the client to rate the level of coincidence of their activities of the past week, according to the intention for each dimension they have identified in the VLQ (0-10). For example, if the client had the intention of an active and close intimate relationship with their partner, did they work toward that intention with their own activity in the past week? If they did nothing at all toward this intention, the activity would be rated zero.

Discrepancies

Together with the client, calculate the discrepancy between the ratings given as to the importance of the valued life dimensions, compared to the ratings given to the coincidence of activities. This difference will show the distance between how the client is acting (activities) and where the client wants to be going (feet and intentions). Ideally, all activities would be moving in the client's intended direction. The dimensions which have the greatest differences should be circled as possible therapeutic goals.

Barriers

Draw a line between the client in the middle and each intention. Pose the question: "What is standing in between you and the intention you have identified?" The client will usually describe the symptom which they came with: pain, tiredness, lack of time, etc. There are usually a few key barriers that are consistently overshadowing all intentions. Have the client write them in the circles in between themselves and their intentions.

Solution

Ask the client: "Is it your belief that the barriers must first be reduced/alleviated before you can go in your intended direction? Is that what you have been doing? Trying to manage or control your symptoms? Is reducing your symptoms your goal here at the clinic?"

Make a new table at the whiteboard/paper where there is room for the clients to explicitly list all of the ways in which he/she has attempted to "manage" the symptoms. Try and organize the client's attempts in terms of functional categories, i.e. according to what function they serve. Are they avoidance strategies? Are they rituals used to distract them from pain? Do the strategies lead to loss of functioning?

Next, ask the clients to make a list of general strategies which he or she has used, and beside this list make two more categories where he/she will describe the results, in both the short and long term, of these strategies. The "short term" results answers the question of whether the symptom was reduced or controlled immediately. The question of "long-term" results is related to the clients described intentions. That is "Did you, by resting, taking pain killers, etc., move closer to your intended directions? Did you come closer to the type of job that you aspire to, or to the social life you want, by resting or taking pain-killers? Repeat the client's intentions when asking these questions about the results of the strategies in the long term. The table could end up looking like this:

What have you tried?	Results	Results	What does this experience tell you?
To manage, control, & reduce symptoms?	*Short term* Were symptoms reduced?	*Long term* Have you come closer to the way you want your life to be?	
Physical therapy	-	-	Didn't work, felt good for the moment
Sick leave	-	-	Didn't work, lost my job
Pain killers	+	-	Didn't work, got dependent on drugs
Rest	-	-	Just got more tired
Avoided physical work	-	-	Got weaker
Alternative therapy	+	-	Just cost a lot of money
Surgery	-	-	Helped at first but then got worse

Table 10.1. Possiblesolutions and results.

3. Creative Hopelessness and Change

Ask the client to examine the results of these strategies/actions while considering valued directions. Then instruct the client to look at the verbal rule "control or manage the pain first" and see if following that rule has brought them closer to, or farther away from, identified valued life directions. Usually, clients will clearly see the futility of their attempts to control pain, but they still have thoughts and feelings that this is the "reasonable" or "logical" thing to do.

Here is an example of a client's "story" about this issue: "Pain and fatigue are blocking most of my attempts to live the way I want to live, and logically, pain and fatigue must be alleviated before I could go back to work or start exercising, or enjoying myself." Here the client shows a "Catch 22," or hopeless situation, wherein his or her emotions say that symptom alleviation must happen before life can go on. But the client's experience shows that attempts to alleviate or control the symptoms only gets them farther away from the way they want to be living. In other words, the client has gotten him/herself "stuck" in attempts to alleviate pain and fatigue which are likely leading him or her in undesirable directions; for example, weight gain, drug dependency, reduced social life, disturbed sleep, impaired ability work.

Take the time to illustrate this, and let the client feel the sense of the futility of the old strategies employed in the service of managing his or her symptoms. Discuss the losses these strategies have incurred, and also the fact that they simply have not worked to alleviate the pain. Let the client feel the "hopelessness" of this situation. Validate the hopelessness of strategies attempting to eliminate symptoms.

Once the client has explored his or her hopelessness, do the following exercise: choose from one of two options, one in which you had no more pain or stress symptoms but none of the other desired life dimensions, or in which you would have as much or more pain, fatigue, and stress symptoms as you do now, but the desired life quality you have described in all of these dimensions. It may be possible to live a life without physical pain (for example, by staying medicated on very high doses of narcotics) but the cost is losing out in all other life dimensions. What direction do you want to move toward? Which option would you choose?

Finally, at the end of session one, choose two or three areas where there are significant discrepancies between the client's "intentions" and his or her activities. Ask the client which dimensions they would choose to work on first, in terms of aligning their activities with their intentions. Then ask them what they intend to do that night, the next day, and the next week, to put their intentions into action. Also address the issue of exposure by making sure that the client understands that in order to move in a valued directions, they must be willing to feel the discomfort of the symptoms they have been working so hard to avoid. Ask them to make a commitment to moving in valued directions even though it means exposure to discomfort.

Session 2: First Group Session

Prepare for this session by drawing a life compass on half of the whiteboard with values written in as in example above. Fill in intentions and barriers in categories exactly as the clients have reported in the first individual session. On the other half write the words "stories" and "but" with room underneath them to write.

Start the group with an uplifting vision of the value to self-realization. Parts of Nelson Mandela's Inauguration speech can be used to highlight the idea that you are obliged to utilize your resources and show your greatness:

Our deepest fear is not that we are inadequate. Our deepest fear is that we are powerful beyond measure. It is our light, not our darkness, that most frightens us. We ask ourselves, "who am I to be brilliant, gorgeous, talented, fabulous?" Actually, who are you NOT to be? You are a child of God. *Your playing small does not serve the world.* There is nothing enlightened about shrinking so that other people won't feel insecure around you. We are born to make manifest the glory of God that is within us. It is not just in some of us, it is in every one. And as we let our light shine, we give others permission to do the same. As we are liberated from our fears our presence liberates others.   – Nelson Mandela

1. Cognitive defusion

Referring back to the whiteboard, ask the clients what happened when they attempted to walk toward their valued directions (not if they succeeded or failed, just what happened). Everything they cite as reasons for not moving in those directions is written on the board under "stories." For example: "I didn't have the strength," "I was too tired," "I was in too much pain," "I couldn't afford it," "I was afraid." The idea of stories is introduced as a way people rationalize why they act in ways that are not consistent with their values.

Tell clients that they are not going to discuss the content of these stories in this group; that is, we will not deal with whether the stories are true or real, but rather we will only look at them as words, and we will consider where those words lead us.

Throughout the rest of this session, whenever clients lapse into "storytelling" in discussing their strategies, the stories are written up on the board but not discussed. As this proceeds, clients will often begin to chuckle at how similar all the stories are and how they all lead in the same direction: avoidance of the pursuit of valued directions. This is addressed lightly however by the therapist: the therapist must never use this to blame, criticize, or coerce the client.

"What is your secret?" exercise

Lead the group in this exercise: "Everyone close your eyes and think about what you least like about yourself. What is it that keeps getting in the way of you achieving the things you want in life? Now, open your eyes. What if I had special glasses and could see what it was you just thought about? How would that feel? Embarrassing? Shameful? Try to think what would be so bad about that secret of yours becoming public? If everyone could see your dark side, what would happen?" Clients then provide their answers, most of which will sound like this: "If people really knew my secret, they wouldn't like me and they would probably leave me."

Next ask the clients to describe what they do to ensure that their secrets stay hidden. Write these strategies up on the board under the heading "Ways of being." Clients give examples of what they do to compensate for their "dark sides" or weaknesses, like "being kind, helping others, pleasing others, being cleaver, being funny." Here the therapist can disclose their own secrets and ways of trying to hide them. As the group shares these secrets they begin to see how similar everyone's secret is. Most vulnerability seems to revolve around the theme of being found worthless, incompetent, or unacceptable, and being rejected as a result. Discuss how these ways of being function as barriers to moving toward valued directions, and contribute to the physiological symptoms clients feels, such as tensed muscles, fatigue, and depression. Throughout this discussion it is important to be open and accepting and to discuss the content that comes up in a defused but not invalidating way.

2. Exposure

At this point in the session, when the clients have applied some basic defusion tactics to their worst "secret," it is valuable to do some exercises to reinforce this. Have the clients imagine a time when their secret became apparent, and in order to hide it they were forced to act in ways that were contrary to their desires, for example, saying yes to something wanted to refuse. This exercise can take the form of a visualization, or a participatory demonstration, like the following:

One therapist plays the client who has worked all day and wants to go home and at 4:45 p.m. Her boss (another therapist) walks in and asks the client to work overtime. The client wants to say no and tries to show that she doesn't want to work by through body language like rubbing her neck, yawning, and avoiding eye contact. The client also makes up some excuses (stories) about why she doesn't want to work late. The boss is very stubborn and does not give up, and finally the client yields and agrees even though she doesn't want to. The scene is then analyzed in terms of what made the client act in ways contradictory to her wishes: e.g., maintaining the "illusion" that she is hard-working, a team player, etc.

Next, do the scene a second time, and have the boss act in the same manner, but the client behaves consistently with her intentions by greeting the boss, making eye contact, showing empathy to the boss's situation, and finally saying "no" to working overtime. Then discuss how the client handled the unpleasant feelings the first and the second time, and which encounter has led to moving in her valued direction. Each client should play the main role here and each scene can be adapted to what types of situations each client has difficulties with. Practicing willingness and defusion skills during the scenes are key: this point is not just to behave effectively, but to feel what you feel, think what you think, AND behave effectively.

End the session by having clients make a commitment to where they are going, how they're going to get there, and how they will confront unpleasant barriers.

Session 3: Second Group Session

Preparation: Draw a life compass, along with values and barriers, on half of the white board. Include as categories the specific intentions and types of barriers the clients have reported. On the other half of the whiteboard write "Stories" and "But." Prepare three to five blank, brightly colored cards for each person and give each participant those cards and a magic marker.

1. Mega visualization

To set the scene for a mega visualization, start off with the funeral exercise. Have the clients close their eyes and imagine they are at their own funeral. They can drift around the room and listen to what people are saying about them: what kind of person they were and how they will be remembered. Then ask the clients to think about what it is they would like people to say about them, and what they wish their legacy to be. What would they want their children to remember? Their spouses? Their colleagues? Their neighbors? What meaning would they want their lives to have, relative to their valued life dimensions? Write these new intentions on the white board.

2. Exercises in cognitive defusion
Exercise one: Fighting or accepting the cards

Begin by asking the group to think about the consequences of trying to make their feet line up with their intentions. Write some examples that they give up on the board, such as: "I couldn't take the time to exercise at night because my husband wanted me at home," or "My boss got angry when I tried to say no." As these stories are generated, write them up on the white board, and ask the client who gave them to write this story on one of the cards they were given. If they have more stories, they should write them down on the extra cards. By the end everyone should have at least three "stories" about why they could not move toward valued directions.

Next, divide clients up in pairs and do two exercises using these cards, demonstrating each exercise before the group begins. For the first exercise, each participant takes the other person's cards and tells the person that they are going to try and throw their cards at them, and that they need to do whatever they can to prevent the cards from landing on them. Each card should be read aloud before it is thrown. The other person should duck the cards, bat them away, etc.

For the second phase of the exercise, the person holding the cards will simply place each card in the other person's lap after they have read it aloud, and the second client can simply observe the card. At the end of this exercise ask the person receiving the cards what the difference was in terms of strain, focus, and attention between the first and second ways of approaching these cards. You should note here that the person did not successfully avoid the cards in either case. Have clients repeat the exercise, with their roles reversed.

A variation on this exercise which can be can be included at this point is one in which one client takes the other's cards and presents them text side out. The other client attempts physically to push the cards away from them, as hard as they can. The other participant should push back equally hard. Next ask the person to simply hold his/her card, with the text toward them, and observe the text. Ask what the difference was in terms of effort and attention. Again it should be noted that in the first scenario, the clients expended a lot of energy trying to resist the cards, but never succeeded in getting rid of them.

Exercise two: Passengers on the bus

Each client takes turns playing the role of the bus driver while the other clients play the roles of the driver's cards, or "passengers." If there are more bus passengers than cards the bus driver can add additional stories like -"I'm especially sensitive to stress," "I have fibromyalgia," of "I need to take care of my family."

The therapist stands in front facing the bus driver, and the passengers stand behind the drivers with their cards. The bus driver faces the values compass and is instructed to drive toward a certain valued intention, for example toward the type of job the person wants. While trying to drive, their passengers come up one by one and try to bully the driver with one of their stories, like "You can't get that job, you don't have the training and you were never good at school, so you can't go back." Another bus passenger might say, "Don't even think about that job, your family needs you to stay home and take care of them." The only way the bus driver can get the passengers to go back and sit down is by offering them compromises on the direction they are moving. A compromise could be that the driver will only work part time, or will settle for a less demanding job. The bus driver may try to reason with each passenger, but the passenger only sits down after negotiating a real compromise in direction.

At the end the bus driver, who is no longer is headed in the valued direction because of all of the compromises she was forced to make, now may stop the bus and try and reason with all of the passengers as to why she wants to go in that direction. But the passengers are stubborn and they just repeat themselves, making the driver tired and more frustrated, and sitting with the bus standing still. The driver then takes the wheel again and to drive toward the valued direction, and this time the passengers walk around the driver bombarding her with their stories and complaints about where she is going. This time, she should try just acknowledging the passengers as they approach, while keeping her own direction in focus.

Everyone in the group should get a turn playing the bus driver. This exercise takes about 45 minutes for 6 people, including some discussion along the way. The points taken from this exercise could be about similarities between the compromises clients made to control or reduce the unpleasant feelings and what the driver has actually done in his or her life. The hopelessness of these compromises should be discussed, along with where these compromises lead and what effect they have or don't have on the unpleasant thoughts and feelings.

3. *Exposure exercises*

Have clients remember back to their darkest secret from the beginning of the session. Take some examples of them from the group, such as "I'm dishonest," or "I'm a failure," and write them on the board. Have them name some situations that elicit these feelings very strongly, then structure a role-playing exposure exercise around one of the scenarios.

The following example is specific to the Swedish client population we worked with in our study, all of whom were on long term sick leave. As part of their disability package, each client has to participate in a "rehab meeting," which is a universally unpleasant experience. In it, they meet with their employer, an insurance company representative, and an occupational therapist. The purpose of the meeting is to assess the client's eligibility for further disability payments.

In this "rehab meeting" exercise each client plays themselves, with therapists and other clients standing in as the other participants. The person who is playing themselves describes for the other role players his or her "nightmare scenario" for the rehab meeting's outcome. In the first dry run of the meeting the client behaves as he or she would do normally. The therapist is with the client playing themselves at all times, and is directing the scene. After the first dry run the role play is analyzed. What direction was the client trying to move in, and what happened to prevent them from doing it?

The second time the scene is played by all the players exactly as before, except the client is given suggestions about how to change the meeting's outcome. Here the therapist makes suggestions as to what types of behavior would move things toward her goal, like putting the other players on her team, writing out a plan beforehand listing what she'd need to do to achieve her desired outcome, taking control of the meeting, and so on.

Clients should also practice showing vulnerability by taking the risk of saying what they really want. For example, the client could say to her employer: "I know I have caused you problems by taking sick leave, and that probably makes you feel that I am unreliable. I cannot say that I'll never take sick leave again, but I can tell you that I care about my job and my colleagues, and that I want my job back." Ask the client what they are risking here. Personal rejection? Professional failure? Validate the client that he is taking a risk by showing vulnerability. Point out however that he is at least betting on a live horse. In the end he may lose, but in betting on the live horse he at least have the option of winning. If he bets on the dead horse and doesn't make his desires known, winning is precluded as an option. At the end of the exercise, end the session by asking each client to make a verbal commitment to use such situations to move toward valued life dimensions.

Session 4: Final Individual Session

The final session involves the same core treatment elements seen before: values, acceptance, defusion, exposure, and commitment. The aim of this session is to allow the client to present his/her life compass with its valued directions rated, and summarize where their feet have been going, what they have been avoiding, and how they will now proceed forward in the directions they most value.

1. Values

The client has worked on identifying his/her life compass in the earlier sessions, and should be able to draw the compass for the therapist. The client should also be able to tell the therapist her intentions in each dimension, as well as give examples of activities that would move her forward. It is important for the therapist to ensure that the activities the client provides as "feet in alignment" for each dimension are actually vital activities, and not just what the client thinks might be appropriate (pliance). The therapist should tell the client that the only way to know if an activity is in alignment with their personal values is by the feeling of the activity elicits in them. For example, a client on sick leave values having an open and sincere relationship with her work colleagues, and an activity she has identified as consistent with that value is visiting them and talking about coming back to work. She has been avoiding them because she thought it would be unpleasant. The only way she will know if this activity of visiting her old job is consistent with her valued direction would be the feeling of vitality in the action. In other words, when the client walks toward her valued direction, she should feel that it is leading her where she wants to go. This is the personal motivation ACT-based therapies use to move clients forward on their own volition. The tasks undertaken in valued dimensions naturally should lead to positive reinforcement. Once the client experiences these natural contingencies, activity in that dimension will increase.

2. Acceptance

By the last session, the client should be able to explain to the therapist why they have been stuck. They should describe what their obstacles have been and what they have been trying to do with those obstacles. The client should demonstrate that they understand what those control strategies led to, and what the alternative strategy of acceptance can do.

It could be a useful idea here for the therapist to play the "mind" of the client as he or she describes what steps he or she intends to take. Before starting the therapist can explain to the client that the future steps and what types of obstacles that the mind produces can be simulated right here and now. The aim of the exercise is to illustrate the workability of different ways of relating to these obstacles: resisting or ignoring on the one hand and acceptance on the other hand. Ask the client to react to his or her own thoughts by physically trying to push them away or trying to ignore them or any other way he or she typically has attempted to "get rid" of these obstacles produced by the mind. The client can pick a step that he or she has chosen to take from the commitments made. An example of this might be that the client is going to go to his or her workplace to ask to get back his or her job, prior to going on disability due to the pain problem. In this exercise, the client will be role playing the step he or she is about to take. In this example, the therapist could set a chair in front of the client and suggest that the client is in the meeting with his or her boss and the boss is sitting in the chair facing the client. The client is asked to try and communicate the message, which he or she has committed to do. The client understands that as he or she is attempting to communicate this message to the boss, the therapist will be "playing the mind" of the client. The therapist can step behind the client and play the most common thoughts which the client has voiced like for example: "you are too old for that", "a person with pain like will never make it, settle for less", "What is your boss doesn't want you back, why take that risk" or "Who do you think you are attempting such a stunt like this, make it easy on yourself, you can have a comfortable carefree life instead".

The job of the client in both parts one and two of this exercise is to try and focus on the commitment made which is to communicate the client's intention of wanting to come back to work to the boss who can help to implement the clients intention. In part one of the exercise, the client illustrates resistance to his or her thoughts played by any means he or she comes up with which is usually arguing with the thoughts, physically trying to push them away, simply ignoring them or doing things to suppress them like talking louder or more aggressively. Just ask the client to note his or her feelings in this first part and the amount of strain, effort and stress this way of relating entailed. In the second part of the exercise, ask the client to practice what he or she has learned about acceptance. Ask the client to pull up a chair next to him or her and make a space for his or her mind (the therapist). The therapist can demonstrate this first if needed. Ask the client to demonstrate what the principles of acceptance would look like in this situation. In most cases the clients demonstrate sitting the "mind" in the chair that he or she has placed close to him or her. The client might put his or her arm around the mind and as the mind babbles warnings of impending risk and catastrophes and ridiculing judgment, the client simply sits close to the mind, looks at the mind occasionally and acknowledges any new thought and returns to the job at hand which in this case is communicating to the boss the clients intentions. After this second part the client is asked how much strain and effort was required in relating his or her unruly thoughts in this part as compared to the first part.

The point of this acceptance exercise is that the client actually experiences the difference between resistance or attempts to ignore and acceptance of the inevitable unpleasant thoughts and feelings that will come as steps are taken in valued directions. Most clients who do this exercise can easily feel that resistance requires significantly more effort and is far more disturbing for the task at hand than is the acceptance way of relating to thoughts and feelings.

3. Exposure/defusion

At this final session the client should be able to demonstrate the principles of using exposure and defusion in simulated situations taken from the committed action plan made in the group session. The principles to be demonstrated here by the client are 1) ability to get into the observing self perspective and see the difference between clean and dirty pain 2) ability to "go into" the experience of pain and fear of pain rather than avoid pain and all that is associated with pain. In this session the client should be able to demonstrate ability to distinguish the pain sensation itself from the thoughts, feelings, and fears associated with the pain and be able to show the skill of going "into" the pain experience and the unpleasant thoughts and feelings associated with the pain, rather than using the previous avoidance strategies. The client should demonstrate an insight stemming from his or her own experience of workability of avoidance versus exposure to these noxious and unpleasant thoughts, feelings and sensations.

Following are some examples of how defusion and exposure can be demonstrated in this last session.

Mindfulness exercises can be used to help the client to "go into" pain rather than avoid it. These exercises are also useful for defusion. Following is an example of how this can be done.

Get yourself comfortable in a sitting position and close your eyes. Begin to focus on your breathing. Try and breathe with your stomach and feel how your belly goes up and down as your body breathes itself with no effort on your part. Feel the sense of your breathing as the center of yourself. Think of your breathing as a way of being in the present. Your breathing makes no judgments, has no associations from the past, makes no warnings of the future, your breathing is in the here and now. You cannot breath from the past or breath for the future. You can only breathe here and now. As you are with your breathing notice the calmness and strength within yourself that comes forward and spreads throughout your whole body.

As you do this, climb into the observer self perspective and simply observe yourself. From this position notice any thoughts or feelings or sensations that come forward and try and get your attention. Most people can start to feel muscle stiffness from sitting still in a position or pain sensations from parts of the body that are usually painful. If your mind starts getting those signals see if you can just notice these messages and go on and keep your focus on your breathing. See if it is possible to receive those pain signals, acknowledge them, and let them be there or pass and return your focus to your breathing and feeling calmness. See if it is possible to have these pain signals yelling at you to get up and get more comfortable or change positions and rather than do what they are telling you, simply acknowledge them and choose to stay where you are and return to your breathing. See what happens to these signals when you choose to stay put.

From the observer position watch how your mind reacts to these pain signals. Watch what kind of pain scripts your mind starts writing for you. It may start telling you that this mindfulness stuff isn't working or remind you of all the other treatments that you have tried that never worked in the real world or it may be warning you right now about all the pending worries, problems or even disasters that are around the corner out there when you stop treatment. Whatever your mind is saying to you, just see if it is possible to notice and acknowledge the thought and return to your breathing. Even if the thought looks very very scary and says terrible things, see if you can regard this thought as a thought, on the same line as all thoughts, look the content of the thought in the face and return to your breathing. These thoughts are natural reactions of your mind to your pain sensations. Notice even your tendencies to want to "deal" with your thoughts. You can feel your urge to want to argue, resist, counteract or obey these thoughts. You can feel the urge to take action to "do something" about these thoughts probably in order to get rid of them. Just see if it is possible to feel these urges and see the counter thoughts produced, acknowledge the workings of your mind and body and see if you can let these be and return to your breathing. In the weeks and months to come practice this exercise several times a day and anytime you start to feel a pain sensation. Sit or stand still and see if you can climb into your observer perspective and just watch what is going on. Give yourself the time and space to observe pain signals and the pain scripts as they are, just sensations and thoughts rather than what they say they are. See if you can be the master rather than become the slave of these phenomena. From the observer self-perspective you have flexibility and choices and can decide yourself what action should be taken. From this perspective you can connect to your own long term valued directions and choose to take steps in those directions while having painful sensations and mischievous thoughts of avoidance and escape. From this perspective you can see that while you have pain, you are not your pain, while you have thoughts and fears associated with these pain sensation, you are much greater than these thoughts and fears. The more you practice this exercise the stronger your observer perspective will be which will lead to more flexibility and freedom to live your life the way you want to live it.

Following is an exposure exercise that can be done in the session and also given to take home to practice.

In this program you have been asked to "go into" your pain experience rather than avoid or escape it. You must have felt much resistance in all kinds of form to this message. We are programmed to "resist" avoid and escape pain and all thoughts of pain. You may have had other such experiences where you are in a scary situation like downhill skiing on a steep hill where your whole body and mind screams "stop" "pull back" but you have learned that the only way to gain control is to actually lean forward into the downhill movement, as scary as that feels. Here is an exercise that we can do here in the session and which you can do at home any time you start to sense your pain coming on. We can take an example here of a recurring headache.

Therapist: Imagine the last time you had a headache. Describe the situation for me.

Client: I had had a very stressful day at the day care center. My whole day seem to be a blur of problems and pressures. From the start, I was late, and rushed like an idiot through all my chores, getting upset at the kids for being so slow, having a fight with my oldest for getting in so late and with Jonas for playing video games so late that he overslept and missed his bus. I skipped my own breakfast and tried to solve the kids' problems and in the end just got angry and left the house yelling which I immediately regretted as soon as I was on my way. When I got to work I went through all the motions of my chores but I was still at home in my thoughts feeling guilty about yelling and wondering about how the kids were doing. Then I felt guilty about not talking to the parents about the problems they were having with their kids as they left them off because I was in my own thoughts. I rushed around all morning trying to solve problems but it didn't matter how much I ran around there were always new problems and it seemed like everyone just demanded and demanded me. On my lunch hour I tried to save time by doing my food shopping so that I could get home earlier. But since I had missed breakfast I felt weak and I started feeling dizzy and my pain starting. I passed a hotdog stand and just stuffed in a greasy hot dog just to stifle my hunger and kept running to get back in time. The afternoon was much the same. We went for an outing in the woods which is something that I normally like to do but I hardly noticed the outdoors because I was so worried about if we had all the food and clothes for each child that I had promised and I was worried about what time each parent was coming today and if we could get to the best spot that I had promised we were to go and get back in time. I was also worried about the weather and if it were to suddenly change, if we really had all the clothes the children would need in that case. Before I knew it, we were back and I had hardly noticed that we had been in the woods and had certainly not enjoyed the experience. I started worrying about dinner and what was going to happen this evening and how I would deal with if Jonas continued to play those video games all night and what was to become of him. I don't even know what we actually did the rest of the afternoon with the children because I was busy worrying about my failure as a mother and seeing Jonas as a destitute marginalized catastrophe. By the time I got home my head was throbbing and I was forced to go to bed which I felt very, very guilty about, but I had no choice.

Therapist: In the story you have told here, how would you describe the way in which you related to the first signals of pain or unpleasant feelings? Try and climb into your observer perspective and describe what you saw in that story.

Client: As I see it now, I disregarded those pain signals until I was forced to yield to them and go to bed.

Therapist: What about the other unpleasant thoughts and feelings? Like the unpleasant worrying about impending disaster like possible change of weather, or yours son's future?

Client: I "got into" those thoughts and obsessed about them. I guess I was trying to solve them in my head in order to get rid of them.

Therapist: When you look at your "obsessing" or trying to mentally solve these future problems how did it effect your day? And if you look at the time you spent on trying to solve those problem, did you solve anything?

Client: No, those thoughts got in the way of me enjoying what I like and I, for sure did not get anywhere with those problem, I just ended up feeling more worried tired and guilty.

Therapist: Here is an exercise we can try here and now to "go into the pain". Let's start back at the beginning of the day where you started feeling pain signals in your neck and shoulders while you were still at home.

You are standing in your kitchen about to up to Jonas and you feel stiffness in your neck and shoulders. Stop there and see if it is possible to climb into the observer perspective and watch yourself. I want you to "go into" those pain signals. See if it is possible to give yourself time and just describe what you see and feel. You may see that as you make space for those pain sensations that they are in constant change. Instead of treating them with irritation, take the time and show them respect and really try to feel and listen to them. Describe out loud what you are feeling. If you have some pain right now in you body you can describe this sensation. You will notice that pain sensations are in constant movement like the ebb and flow of the ocean. If you rotate your head and shoulders gently around those painful spots you will notice that you influence the sensations. Try and listen to what these sensations are telling you. Instead of regarding these sensations as a nuisance, see if it is possible to show compassion towards these sensations and see if you can understand what they are trying to tell you. Your body has a fantastic alarm system that sends pain signals as messengers and tells you that something is the matter, something is out of balance. What do you think that stiffness and pain from you neck and shoulders is trying to tell you?

Client: As I see it now, it is telling me that I woke up with tenseness and I should have taken the time to stretch, instead of rushing out of bed. It is telling me to do that now, rather than rush up to Jonas and try to solve his video game problem. It is asking me to sit down and take the time to relax and eat breakfast and prepare myself for my day. It is saying that I need to see to my own needs before I can help others with their needs.

Therapist: If that small pain sensation said all those words of wisdom to you in that short span of time, think of all the answers you have within yourself, if you just took the time to listen. Isn't is wonderful to see that your body tells you when you are out of balance and it tells you how to act in order to take care of yourself properly to get in balance again.

Homework exercise

Try and see your pain signals no matter how small. They may be a red flag signaling you to stop what you are doing so give yourself time and space to stop, feel, describe and listen to your pain. See if it is possible to see your pain as your teacher. Let the pain in and make space for it. Let the pain fill your senses and describe it to yourself. Listen to its message fully. When you are satisfied that you have fully felt and understood the message, step up and do what needs to be done in order to regain your balance and take steps in vital directions. Try to write down the whole "pain chain": the context, the actual pain sensation, the script the mind creates as a reaction to the pain sensation, your urges to "alleviate" the pain and what steps you choose to take which you know are consistent with your valued direction.

4. Commitment

At the end of this last session the client is asked to make a commitment with regard to taking steps in valued directions as well as sticking with the behavior required in these directions with persistency even in the face of the inevitable difficulties life serves up. In this session the therapist goes back to the life compass which the client filled out from the first session and reexamines the commitments made in vital directions from the 10 dimensions of life. Considering all the work that the client has done in this program: identification of valued directions (vitality), experience of diffusion and exposure, what commitments is the client willing to make towards living the vital life he or she wants to live AND have the inevitable noxious pain sensations, discomfort and negative thoughts associated with that pain.

During the time of the 4 week program, the client has experienced taking steps as well as what types of obstacles have come forward and tried to stop this progress. The client might have also experienced that the steps he or she believed would be alignment with his or her values turned out, in fact, not to be. For example, one client took a step towards going back to work but when doing this discovered that there were many more options open to her. By going back to work and speaking with her boss she discovered that she was qualified to start in a continuing education program that would bring her closer to her interest of teaching in special education. Her previous "intention" with regard to work was consistent "working with children in such a way that I would contribute with what I can do best in a creative way that helps me also develop as a person" but the steps she thought would bring her closer to this intention changed as they always will. She changed her commitment from "going back to my old job" to now starting the continuing education program. This example will help the client to realize that while the valued direction is fairly consistent regardless of life changes, conditions and age, the steps one takes to be consistent with those directions will always vary.

The client is asked how he or she will know if a step he or she commits to is consistent or not with the set course in valued direction. Examples can be taken from the client's life where he or she made choices and mindfulness exercises can be used to help the client to be able to make the distinction between, vital or non-vital, living or dead. Most clients have experienced making decisions for non-vital reasons, for example because someone else wanted you to do something. Most clients know the feeling of going through the motions of an activity because they were forced to or felt that had no other choice. The feeling of doing something under coercion is a very non-vital feeling. This can be compared to the very different feeling of taking a step in a direction that you have dreamed of going. Mindfulness can be used here to help the client feel in all senses what this difference is. The client is invited to use this feeling of vitality as the measure by which to evaluate whether steps taken are indeed vital (in alignment with valued direction) or not. In some ways this is an "either or" call. You are either in your direction, your course or out of your course. You may be far away and still be in your course of direction. If you have ever been involved in navigation, you know that you set your course when you know where you want to go and you need to keep checking your compass or GPS to see if you are still on course. In this case the GPS will be your feeling of vitality. In order to feel vitality, you will need to stop, get present to what you are doing and how you are feeling and make an evaluation, if the steps you are taking are vital or non-vital, living or dead. These answers can only be found within yourself.

At the end of the session the client is asked to state and write down commitments in the form of steps that he or she is now willing to take in valued directions along with what activities which will be required in taking those steps.

Impact of this Protocol

This protocol was evaluated in a small randomized controlled trial described by Dahl et al. (2004). A random sample of 24 persons was approached from among a pool of 220 chronic pain patients working in public sector jobs who had missed work repeatedly over the last year due to pain, but continued to work. Using this sample the present ACT protocol (N = 11) was compared to medical treatment as usual (MTAU; N = 8). The four ACT sessions were delivered weekly. Follow up occurred six months later. The results were striking. During the six month follow up, MTAU participants visited their physician 15.1 times on average; ACT participants visited the doctor at an 87% lower rate: 1.9 visits on average during follow-up. Work related absences were even more dramatic. During the six month follow up MTAU workers missed 56.1 days of work on average; ACT participants missed work at a 99% lower rate: .5 missed days on average during follow-up.

How to Scale this Approach into More Extensive Protocols

The same basic approach described here can be scaled into pain interventions of any scope and length. The McCracken et al. (in press) protocol mentioned earlier provides a concrete model that also shows how many of the procedures more commonly used in pain programs can be integrated into an ACT model.

In this program treatment was residential or even hospital based and lasted three to four weeks. Physiotherapists, occupational therapists, nurses, physicians, and psychologists all worked together applying a program that was ACT based. Treatment was always conducted in a group format, five days per week, approximately six hours a day.

Some of the same services that are typically part of in-patient pain programs were part of this program. For example, physical exercise groups involved graded exposure and movement and occurred twice daily. Similarly, health habits and occupational skills were addressed much as they might be in any pain unit. Daily relaxation training sessions taught clients to be sensitive to muscular tension and to learn to let go of physical effort. What was different was that ACT treatment principles permeated these components. For example, the program attempted to undermine the causal role of thoughts and feelings, and address the unhelpful nature of struggling with the form or thoughts and feelings as a method of producing progress. Action or inaction was addressed instead as a matter of choice and workability. These components were included even in physical therapy and occupational therapy elements. For example, movement was not cast primarily as a means of feeling better but of living better. Similarly, relaxation was not presented as a means of fighting anxiety, but as a means of learning to let go.

Psychology groups were also held daily, and served as a hub of the ACT model. In the contexts of choosing meaningful directions in life, patients were asked to look at the effectiveness of pain control and reduction strategies. Patients were taught to be more aware of their emotions on the one hand, but to make more room for difficult thoughts and feelings related to their lives and the role of pain in it on the other. Mindfulness mediation exercises were used and practices regularly. Sensation focusing exercises helped patients experience directly that activity and even enjoyment was possible, even when pain was present. Relaxation exercises were practices as well, but always aimed at bodily awareness and improvement of functioning, not escape from feelings. More behavioral methods such as habit reversal were also used. No cognitive restructuring exercises or cognitive disputation procedures were used anywhere in the protocol. The goal was not changing thoughts and feelings, it was engaging in valued actions.

This program produced notable improvements. The average time from initial assessment to admission to the program was 4 months; the times from admission to release and follow up was also 4 months. The amount of change from initial assessment to admission and from admission to follow-up could thus be compared. 108 patients with chronic pain averaging over 10 years duration were treated. The results are shown below. On virtually every measure, much larger changes were found when the ACT protocol was implemented. McCracken also showed that many of these changes co-varied with changes in the acceptance of pain as measured by the CPAQ, particularly improvements in psychosocial disability, timed sitting and standing, depression, anxiety, and physical disability.

Conclusion

These two protocols vary widely, but there are both thoroughly consistent with an ACT model. One protocol leads with values rather than acceptance; while the other leads with acceptance and works to values. One includes extensive use of mindfulness and relaxation techniques (the latter carefully cast as "letting go" rather then "winning the struggle"), while the other uses these elements only in a limited way. One is a multi-disciplinary, multi-element program, while the other is targeted. Yet they are both ACT.

Making contact with one's true values almost always leads immediately to pain, be it physiological or psychological. This is a lot to ask of anyone, and without the behavioral flexibility that comes with acceptance, and defusion, it can seem like an unreasonable request. Acceptance and defusion are necessary before client values can be fully utilized. Conversely, acceptance and defusion are not ends in themselves – they are important precisely because they enable valued actions. Thus, whether you begin with values or you begin with acceptance and defusion you end

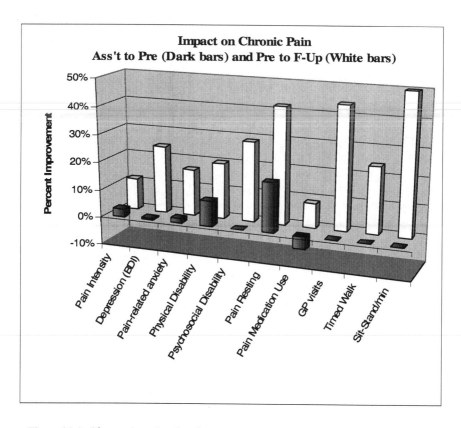

Figure 10.2. Changes in pain related measures from initial assessment to pre-assessment (average length of time in between = 3.9 months) and from pre-assessment to follow-up (average length of time in between = 3.9 months) in the McCracken et al. (in press) study.

up in much the same spot. Whether either is better empirically is not yet known, but in terms of processes they are both ACT protocols.

ACT is not a technology, although in contains technology. ACT is an approach. The two protocols described here are but two of many specific ACT pain protocols that might be constructed for specific purposes and contexts. What prevents chaos is that the model is quite specific about the targets, processes, and purposes of ACT interventions.

Chapter 11

Elisabeth with an ACT Alternative

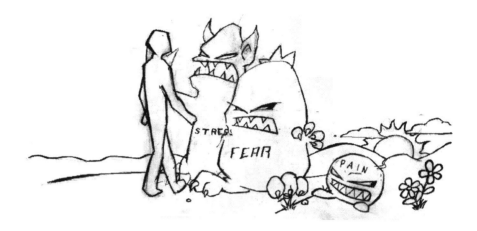

And so we return to Elisabeth, as she looks at her life in a different way.

"When I stood back and looked at my life on that whiteboard I started to cry. I saw so clearly that I was so far away from where I wanted to be. When I called the health center and tried to get help, I expected that they were going to help me get rid of my pain and help me manage my stress better. I don't think I have talked to anyone about my hopes and dreams about life for the past 20 years. Not since I used to meet my friends and we would talk about our dreams. It was just choking to see my life laid out that clearly on that whiteboard. It was also very sad to see that even though I was working from dawn to late at night, every day of the week without rest, I was only getting further and further away from where I wanted to go in my life. It was like I was digging my own grave. The harder I dug the deeper I got away from life."

"I really felt sorrowful about this. The therapist didn't try to comfort me or tell me that things would get better. In fact, she agreed with me that this was a sad, sad story. After awhile I asked her what I could do? I asked her if she knew what the answer was. She never gave me any answers but asked me if I was willing to let the rope go and stop fighting with the monster. She was referring to the monster story. She asked me to look at those stories and how I had fought them and what was my experience of what they had led to. She asked if I was willing to let that fight go. She asked if I wanted to reclaim my life and get closer to those dreams I had."

"The thought of getting my life back and pursuing my dreams filled me with a chilling fear but also excitement at the mere possibility. I told her yes, I would love nothing more than to do that BUT ... and then I realized that the same old stories came up even when I just allowed myself to dream. We both laughed at how those stories come up at the mere thought of doing what I wanted, let alone actually doing them. The therapist asked me to take a few examples of my intentions that I had written and asked me what my 'feet' could do if they were my intentions. That wasn't hard. I have thought of what I would do, many, many times. I have thought of, for example, going on that evening course for special education that is being offered now. I have thought of calling my old friends and suggesting that we meet for coffee downtown on Friday like we used to. I saw that my old sports club was organizing aerobics in the school right near where I live. I thought that would be fun to go to. I always knew what I wanted to do, I just never followed through with it. The therapist asked why I didn't follow through and we laughed because it was the same old 'stories' that popped up and stopped me. When I saw that, I knew what she meant and I knew what I needed to do. I was going to start doing what I wanted to be doing and not let those 'stories' get into the drivers seat of my life. I told her that I intended to reclaim my life starting now. She looked at me and said, Elisabeth, I want to join you in that effort."

"It is a scary thought to think that you can do what you want in your life. It was, in fact, easier to let my 'stories' take over because then I had a good excuse for not going after my dreams. It is really easy to avoid dreams by giving these excuses. It is easier to be small than to stick your neck out and be big. I don't understand why it is easier for people around you to listen to excuses than it to listen to what you really want. People seem to recognize excuses and stories."

"Like last week when my boss asked me if I wanted to go on this course for special education. I said like I usually say that I would really like to do that but I just can't leave my family and responsibilities one evening a week every week for a whole semester. My boss seemed to really understand that and went off to ask someone else. If I had said instead, 'that is exactly what I want to do and I am having the thought that I can't leave my family' my boss would not have known what to say. It's like you are supposed to be clear about yes or no. But for me I feel both yes and no at the same time."

"I thought that those 'stories' warning me about failures should be taken seriously, more seriously than what I wanted. Now I know that if I don't take what I want seriously, I will loose my life as I already have to a great degree. I kept my life compass with me and kept looking at it until it was in my head. Somehow opportunities just came up in one way or another that I saw and acted upon according to my 'compass'."

"For example, while I was in the grocery store, I met one of my old friends. Before I would have avoided her because I would have been afraid that she would want to meet and I knew I had no time for that. But this time I walked right towards her and told her how much I had missed her and our group of friends. I suggested that we meet this Friday. She seemed as happy as I was about the idea of meeting again. Maybe she had been doing the same thing as I had been doing, avoiding social contacts."

"Things like that just kept happening. I ran into an old soccer friend and she told me she was going to that aerobics class that I have seen in the paper. She said it was great and that if I came the next evening, she would meet me outside and show me what I had missed. Life just opened up again, but not without problems. As my feet go in these directions that I want to go, all the old 'stories' come back. They can be very convincing. Sometimes they win over me."

"Other people in my life said things that were similar to my own stories. When I told my mother-in-law that I had signed up for an evening course, she said that I should save my energy for taking care of my family. But then I realized that I had also let others get into my drivers seat instead of my own wishes."

"When I let go of that rope, and stopped fighting with the monster, I had a lot more energy to get my feet in the direction I wanted to go. This is the strange part. Even though I did as much and more than I did before, I felt much more satisfied. I have just as much pain or more, felt stressed and tired but I felt more in tune with myself."

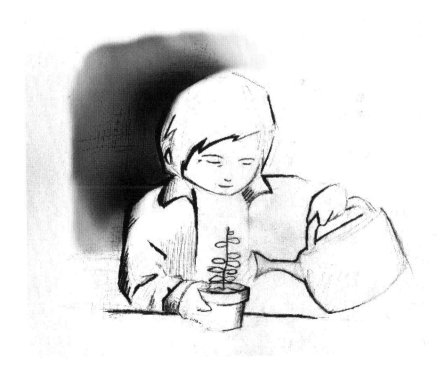

Conclusion

This book has not been intended so much as a how-to-do-it manual but rather a description of principles behind a particular approach, functional analysis and treatment as applied to individuals who have gotten stuck in chronic pain and stress symptoms. The hypothesis suggested as to why individuals get stuck is that vital life dimensions get put on hold in the service of managing the symptoms and life quality is subsequently reduced. The functional analysis is the life-line the therapist needs to go into therapy with the client. The therapeutic alliance between the therapist and the client is of utmost importance. The client's values constitute the context of the therapy and exposure is the main therapeutic element.

Following is a summary of the main principles of the ACT model as described in this book.

- Most difficulties of being stuck in pain and stress have to do with avoidance and attempts to control, manage, or eliminate these symptoms of the other experiences they engender.
- Psychological avoidance of pain and stress have to do with cognitive fusion and its various effects.
- Clients are not broken, and in the areas of acceptance and defusion they have the psychological resources they need, if these can be harnessed.
- To take a new direction, we must let go of an old one. If the problem with pain and stress is chronic, the client's solutions are probably part of them.
- Some verbal rules create "stuckness", believe in your experience.
- The value of any action is its workability measured against the client's true values. The bottom line issue is living well with feelings of pain and stress, not living pain and stress- free life.
- Two things are needed to transform the situation and reclaim your life: accept and move.

References

Aarflot, T., & Bruusgaard, D. (1994). Chronic musculoskeletal complaints and subgroups with special reference to uric acids. *Scandinavian Journal of Rheumatology, 23,* 25-29.

Abbott, J., & Berry, N. (1991). Returning to work during the year following first myocardial infarction. *British Journal of Medicine, 30,* 268-270.

Alaranta, H., Rytökoski, U., Rissanen, A., Talo, S., Rönnemaa, T., Puukka, P., et al. (1994). Intensive physical and psychosocial training for patients with back pain: A controlled clinical trial. *Spine, 19,* 339-49.

Allen, D., & Waddell, G. (1989). A historical perspective on low back pain and disability. *Orthopedic Scandinavia Supplement, 234,* 1-23.

Altmaier, E., Lehman, T., Russell, D., Weinstein, J., & Feng Kao, C. (1992). The effectiveness of psychological interventions for the rehabilitation of low back pain. A randomized controlled trial evaluation, *Pain, 49,* 329-335.

Andersson, G., (1997) The epidemiology of spinal disorders. In J. Frymoyer (Ed.), *The adult spine: Principles and practice* (2nd ed., pp. 93-141). New York: Raven Press.

Andersson, H., Ejlertsson, G., Leden, I., & Rosenberg, C. (1993). Chronic pain in a geographical population: studies of differences in age, gender, social class and pain localization. *Clinical Journal of Pain, 9,* 174-182.

Arbus, L., Fajadet, B., Aubert, D., Morre, M., & Goldberger, E. (1990). Activity of tetrazepam (myolastan) in low back pain: A double blind trial versus placebo. *Journal of Clinical Trials, 27,* 258-67.

Arkuszewski, Z. (1986). The efficacy of manual treatment in low back pain: A clinical trial. *Manual Medicine, 2,* 68-71.

Aronson, M. (1997). Nonsteroidal anti-inflammatory drugs, traditional opioids and tramadol: Contrasting therapies for the treatment of chronic pain. *Clinical Therapy, 19,* 420-432.

Aronsson, G., Gustavsson, K., & Dallner, M. (2000). Sick but yet at work: An empirical study of sickness presenteeism. *Epidemiology Community Health, 54,* 502-509.

Asfour, S., Khlil, T., Waly, S., Goldberg, M., Rosomoff, R., & Rosomoff, H. (1990). Biofeedback in back muscle strengthening. *Spine, 15,* 510-513.

Aube, J., Fleury, J., & Smetana, J. (2000). Changes in women's roles: Impact on social policy, implications for the mental health of women and children. *Development and Psychopathology, 12,* 633-656.

Barlow, D., Craske, M., Cerny, J., & Klosko, J. (1989). Behavioral treatment of panic disorder. *Behavior Therapy, 20,* 261-282.

Beck, A. T., Rush, A. J., Shaw, B. F., & Emery, G. (1979). *Cognitive therapy of depression.* New York: Guilford.

Bendix, A., Bendix, R., Vaegter, K., Lund, C., Frölund, L., & Holm, L. (1996). Multidisciplinary intensive treatment for chronic low back pain: A randomized, prospective study. *Cleveland Clinical Journal of Medicine, 63,* 62-69.

Bendix, A., Bendix, T., Labriola, M., & Boekgaard, P. (1998). Functional restoration for chronic low back pain: Two year follow-up of two randomized clinical trials. *Spine, 23,* 717-25.

Bennet, R. (1999). Emerging concepts in the neurobiology of chronic pain: Evidence of abnormal sensory processing in fibromyalgia. *Mayo Clinical Proceedings, 74,* 385-398.

Bennet, R., Clark, S., & Walczyk, J. (1998). A randomized double blind placebo-controlled study of growth hormone in the treatment of fibromyalgia. *American Journal of Medicine, 104,* 227-231.

Berry, H., Bloom, B., & Hamilton, E. (1982). Naproxen sodium, diflinisal and placebo in the treatment of chronic back pain. *Annals of Rheumatic Disorders, 41,* 129-132.

Beurskens, A., de Vet, H., Köke, A., Lindeman, E., Regtop, W., van der Heijden, G., et al. (1995). Efficacy of traction for non-specific low back pain: A randomized clinical trial. *Lancet, 346,* 1596-1600.

Beurskens, A., van der Heijden, G., de Vet, H., Köke, A., & Lindeman, E. et al. (1995). The efficacy of traction for lumbar back pain: Design of a randomized clinical trial. *Journal of Manipulative Physiological Therapeutics, 18,* 141-147.

Bigos, S., Battie, M. C., Spengler, D. M., Fisher, L. D., Fordyce, W. E., Hansson, T. H., et al. (1991). A prospective study of work perceptions and psychosocial factors affecting the report of back injury. *Spine, 16,* 1-6.

Bigos, S., Bowyer, O., Braen, A., Brown, K., Deyo, R., & Haldeman, S. (1994). Acute low-back problems in adults. *Clinical practice guidelines.* 14. (AHCPR Publication No. 95-0642). Rockville, MD: Agency for Health Care Policy and Research, Public Health Service, US.

Boden, S., Davis, D., Dina, T., Patronas, N., & Wiesel, S. (1990). Abnormal magnetic resonance scans of the lumbar spine in asymptomatic subjects. *Journal of Bone Joint Surgery, 72,* 403-408.

Bond, F. (2004). ACT for stress. In S. C. Hayes & K. D. Strosahl (Eds.), *A practical guide to Acceptance and Commitment Therapy* (pp. 275-294). New York: Kluwer/Plenum.

Bond, F. W., & Bunce, D. (2000). Mediators of change in emotion-focused and problem-focused worksite stress management interventions. *Journal of Occupational Health Psychology, 5,* 156-163.

Bond, F., & Hayes, S. C. (2002). ACT at work. In F. Bond & W. Dryden (Eds.), *Handbook of brief cognitive behavior therapy* (pp. 117-140). Chichester, England: Wiley.

Boos, N., Reider, R., Schade, V., Spratt, K., Semmer, N., & Aebi, M. (1995). The diagnostic accuracy of magnetic resonance imaging, work perception and psychosocial factors in identifying symptomatic disc herniation. *Spine, 20,* 2613-2625.

Borenstein, D., O'Mara, J., Boden, S., Lauerman, W., Jacobson, A., Platenberg, C., et al. (1998). *A 7 year follow-up study of the value of lumbar spine MR to predict the development of low back pain in asymptomatic individuals.* Poster, ISSLS, Brussels.

Borkovec, T. D., & Hu, S. (1990). The effect of worry on cardiovascular response to phobic imagery. *Behaviour Research and Therapy, 28,* 69-73.

Borkovec, T. D., Lyonfields, J. D., Wiser, S. L., & Diehl, L. (1993). The role of worrisome thinking in the suppression of cardiovascular response to phobic imagery. *Behaviour Research and Therapy, 31,* 321-324.

Brage, S., Nygård, J., & Tellnes, G. (1998). The gender gap in musculoskeletal-related long-term sickness in Norway. *Scandinavian Journal of Social Medicine, 26,* 34-43.

Branthaver, B., Stein, G. F., & Mehran A. (1995) Impact of a medical back care program on utilization of services and primary care physician satisfaction in a large, multispecialty group practice health maintenance organization. *Spine, 10,* 1165-1169.

Brattberg, G. (1993). Back pain and headache in Swedish schoolchildren; a longitudinal study. *The Pain Clinic, 6,* 157-162.

Brattberg, G. (1994). The incidence of back pain and headache among Swedish schoolchildren. *Quality of Life Research, 67,* 29-34.

Breivik, H., Hesla, P., Molnar, I., & Lind, B. (1976). Treatment of chronic low back pain and sciatica: Comparison of caudal epidural injections of bupivacaine and methylprednisolone with bupivacaine followed by saline. *Advances in Pain Research and Therapy, 1,* 927-932.

Bruder-Mattson, S. F., & Hovanitz, C. A. (1990). Coping and attributional styles as predictors of depression. *Journal of Clinical Psychology, 46,* 557-565.

Burton, A., Symonds, T., Zinzen, E., Tillotson, K., Caboor, D., Van Roy, P., et al. (1997). Is ergonomic intervention alone sufficient to limit musculoskeletal problems in nurses? *Occupational Medicine, 47,* 25-32.

Bush, C., Ditto, B., & Feuerstein, M. (1985). A controlled evaluation of paraspinal EMG biofeedback in the treatment of chronic low back pain. *Health Psychology, 4,* 307-321.

Bush C., & Hillier, S. (1991). A controlled study of caudal epidural injections of triamcinolone plus procaine for the management of intractable sciatica. *Spine, 16,* 572-575.

Carette, S., Leclaire, R., Marcoux, S., Morin, F., Blaise, G., St.-Pierre, A., et al. (1997). Epidural corticosteroid injections for sciatica due to herniated nucleus pulposus. *New England Journal of Medicine, 336,* 1634-1640.

Carlsson, C-A., & Nachemson, A. (2000). Hur uppstår smärta-ryggsmärtans neurofysiologi [What is the process of back pain's neurophysiology]. In *Ont i ryggen, ont i nacken [Pain in back, pain in neck],* vol. I (pp. 265-290). Stockholm: SBU.

Clark, D. M., Ball, S., & Pape, A. (1991). An experimental investigation of thought suppression. *Behaviour Research and Therapy, 29,* 253-257.

Clauw, D. (1997). Fibromyalgia: More than just a just a musculoskeletal disease. *American Family Physician, 52,* 843-851.

Coan, R. M., Wong, G., Ku, S. L., Chan, Y. C., Wang, L., Ozer, F. T., et al. (1980). The acupuncture treatment of low back pain: A randomized controlled study. *Annual Journal of Chinese Medicine, 8,* 181-189.

Cooper, M. L., Russell, M., Skinner, J. B., Frone, M. R., & Mudar, P. (1992). Stress and alcohol use: Moderating effects of gender, coping, and alcohol expectancies. *Journal of Abnormal Psychology, 101,* 139-152.

Cuckler, J. M., Bernini, P. A., Weisel, S., Booth, R. E., Rothman, R. H., & Pickens, G. T. (1985). The use of steroids in the treatment of lumbar radicular pain. *Journal of Bone and Joint Surgery, 67*(1), 63-66.

Cutler, R., Fishbain, D., Rosomoff, H., Abdel-Moty, E., Khalil, T., & Rosomoff, R. (1994). Does nonsurgical pain center treatment of chronic pain return patients to work? *Spine, 19,* 643-652.

Dahl, J., Wilson, K. G., & Nilsson, A. (2004). Acceptance and Commitment Therapy and the treatment of persons at risk for long-term disability resulting from stress and pain symptoms: A preliminary randomized trial. *Behavior Therapy, 35,* 785-802.

Dautzenberg, M., Diederiks, J., Philipsen, H., & Tan, F. (1999). Multigenerational care giving and well-being: Distress of middle-aged daughters providing assistance to elderly parents. *Women and Health, 29,* 57-74.

Dawkins, R. (1982). *The extended phenotype.* New York: Freeman.

DeGenova, M. K., Patton, D. M., Jurich, J. A., & MacDermid, S. M. (1994). Ways of coping among HIV-infected individuals. *Journal of Social Psychology, 134,* 655-663.

Deyo, R., Walsh, N., Martin, D., Schoenfeld, L., & Ramamurthy, S. (1990). A controlled trial of transcutaneous electrical nerve stimulation (TENS) and exercise for chronic low back pain. *New England Journal of Medicine, 322,* 1627-1634.

Donaldson, S., Romney, D., Donaldson, M., & Skubick, D. (1994). Randomized study of the application of single motor unit biofeedback training to chronic low back pain. *Journal of Occupational Rehabilitation, 4,* 23-37.

Donchin, M., Woolf, O., Kaplan, L., & Floman, Y. (1990). Secondary prevention of low back pain. A clinical trial. *Spine, 15,* 1317-1320.

Edelist, G., Gross, A., & Langer, F. (1976). Treatment of low back pain with acupuncture. *Canadian Anaesiology Society Journal, 23,* 303-306.

Eifert, G. H., & Heffner, M. (2003). The effects of acceptance versus control contexts on avoidance of panic-related symptoms. *Journal of Behavior Therapy and Experimental Psychiatry, 34,* 293-312.

Einaggar, I., Nordin, M., Sheikhzadeh, A., Parnianpour, M., & Kahanovitz, N. (1991). Effects of spinal flexion and extension exercises on low-back pain and spinal mobility in chronic mechanical low-back pain patients. *Spine, 16,* 967-972.

Englund, L. (2000). Sick-listing-attitudes and doctors' practice, with special emphasis on sick-listing in primary health care. *Acta Universitatis Upsaliensis.* Comprehensive Summaries of Uppsala Dissertations from the Faculty of Medicine, 965-997, Uppsala, ISBN 91-554-4811-9.

Evans, D., Burke, M., Lloyd, K., Roberts, E., & Roberts, G. (1978). Lumbar spinal manipulation on trial, Part 1: Clinical assessment. *Rheumatology and Rehabilitation, 17,* 46-53.

Flor, H., & Birbaumer, N. (1993). Comparison of the efficacy of electromyographic biofeedback, cognitive behavior therapy and conservative interventions in the treatment of chronic musculoskeletal pain. *Journal of Consulting and Clinical Psychology, 61,* 653-658.

Flor, H., Fydrich, T., & Turk, D. (1992). Efficacy of multidisciplinary pain treatment centers: A meta-analytic review. *Pain, 49,* 221-223.

Foa, E. B., & Riggs, D. S. (1995). Post-traumatic stress disorder following assault: Theoretical considerations and empirical findings. *Current Directions in Psychological Science, 4,* 61-65.

Folkesson, H., Larsson, B., & Tegle, S. (1993). *Health Care and social services in seven European countries,* SOS rapport, 6. Stockholm: Social Health and Welfare Department.

Fordyce, W. (1976). *Behavioral Methods for Chronic Pain and Illness.* St. Louis, MO: Mosby.

Fordyce, W., Brockway, J., Bergman, J., & Spengler, D. (1986). Acute back pain: A control group comparison of behavioral versus traditional management methods. *Journal of Behavioral Medicine, 9,* 127-140.

Fox, R., Rotatori, A. F., Macklin, F., & Green, H. (1983). Assessing reinforcer preference in severe behaviorally disordered children. *Early Child Development & Care, 11,* 113-121.

Frost, H., Klaber Moffett, J. A., Moser, J. S., & Fairbank, J. C. T. (1995). Randomised controlled trial for evaluation of fitness programme for patients with chronic low back pain. *British Medical Journal, 310,* 151-154.

Geiser, D. (1992). *A comparison of acceptance-focused and controlled focused psychological treatments in a chronic pain treatment center.* (Doctoral dissertation, University of Nevada, Reno, 1992). Dissertation Abstracts International, B 54/02, 1096.

Gibson, T., Grahame, R., Harkness, J., Woo, P., Blagrave, P., & Hills, R. (1985). Controlled comparison of short-wave diathermy treatment with osteopathic treatment in non-specific low-back pain. *Lancet, 8440,* 1258-1261.

Gold, D. B., & Wegner, D. M. (1995). Origins of ruminative thought: Trauma, incompleteness, nondisclosure, and suppression. *Journal of Applied Social Psychology, 25,* 1245-1261.

Goodkin, K., Gullion, C., & Agras, S. (1990). A randomized, double blind, placebo controlled trial of trazodone hydrochloride in chronic low back pain syndrome. *Journal of Clinical Psychopharmacology, 10,* 269-278.

Gregg, J. (2004). *Development of an acceptance-based treatment for the self-management of diabetes.* Unpublished doctoral dissertation, University of Nevada, Reno.

Grossi, G., Soares, J., Angesleva, J., & Perski, A. (1999). Psychosocial correlates of long-term sick-leave among patients with musculoskeletal pain. *Pain, 80,* 607-619.

Gunn, C., Milbrandt, W., Little, A., & Mason, K. (1980). Dry needling of muscle motor points for chronic low back pain: a randomized clinical trial with long term follow-up. *Spine, 5,* 279-291.

Gutiérrez, O., Luciano, C., Rodríguez, M., & Fink, B. C. (2004). Comparison between an acceptance-based and a cognitive-control-based protocol for coping with pain. *Behavior Therapy, 35,* 767-784.

Haldorsen, E., Kronholm, K., Skouen, J., & Ursin, H. (1998). Multimodal cognitive-behavioral treatment for patients sicklisted for musculoskeletal pain: A randomized controlled study. *Scandinavian Journal of Rheumatology, 27,* 16-25.

Hamberg, K., Johannsson, E., Lindgren, G., & Westman, G., (1997). The impact of marital relationship on the rehabilitation process in a group of women with longstanding musculoskeletal disorders. *Scandinavian Journal of Social Medicine, 13,* 498-503.

Hansen, F., Bendix, T., Skov, P., Jensen, C. V., Kristensen, J. H., Krohn, L., et al. (1993). Intensive, dynamic back-muscle exercises, conventional physiotherapy, or placebo-control treatment of low-back pain: A randomized, observer- blind trial. *Spine, 18*(1), 98-108.

Harkapaa, K., Jarvikoski, A., Mellin, G., & Hurri, H. (1989). A controlled study on the outcome of inpatient and outpatient treatment of low-back pain. Part I. *Scandinavian Journal of Rehabilitation Medicine, 21,* 81-89.

Harkapaa, K., Mellin, G., Jarvikoski, A., & Hurri, H. (1990). A controlled study on the outcome of inpatient and outpatient treatment of low-back pain. Part III. *Scandinavian Journal of Rehabilitation Medicine, 22,* 181-188.

Hayes, S. C. (1993). Analytic goals and the varieties of scientific contextualism. In S. C. Hayes, L. J. Hayes, H. W. Reese, & T. R. Sarbin (Eds.), *Varieties of scientific contextualism* (pp. 11-27). Reno, NV: Context Press.

Hayes, S. C. (2004). Acceptance and Commitment Therapy, Relational Frame Theory, and the third wave of behavioral and cognitive therapies. *Behavior Therapy, 35,* 639-665.

Hayes, S. C., Barnes-Holmes, D., & Roche, B. (Eds.). (2001). Relational Frame Theory: A Post-Skinnerian account of human language and cognition. New York: Plenum Press.

Hayes, S. C., Bissett, R., Korn, Z., Zettle, R. D., Rosenfarb, I., Cooper, L., et al. (1999). The impact of acceptance versus control rationales on pain tolerance. *The Psychological Record, 49,* 33-47.

Hayes, S. C., Bissett, R., Roget, N., Padilla, M., Kohlenberg, B. S., Fisher, G., et al. (2004). The impact of acceptance and commitment training and multicultural training on the stigmatizing attitudes and professional burnout of substance abuse counselors. *Behavior Therapy, 35,* 821-835.

Hayes, S. C., & Smith, S. (in press). *Out of your mind and into your life: The new Acceptance and Commitment Therapy*. Oakland, CA: New Harbinger.

Hayes, S. C., & Strosahl, K. D. (Eds.). (2005). *A practical guide to Acceptance and Commitment Therapy*. New York: Springer-Verlag.

Hayes, S. C., Strosahl, K., & Wilson, K. G. (1999). *Acceptance and Commitment Therapy: An experiential approach to behavior change*. New York: Guilford Press.

Hayes, S. C., Strosahl, K. D., Wilson, K. G., Bissett, R. T., Pistorello, J., Toarmino, D., et al. (2004). Measuring experiential avoidance: A preliminary test of a working model. *The Psychological Record, 54*, 553-578.

Hayes, S. C., & Wilson, K. G. (1993). Some applied implications of a contemporary behavior-analytic view of verbal events. *The Behavior Analyst, 16*, 283-301.

Hayes, S. C., & Wilson, K. G. (1994). Acceptance and Commitment Therapy: Altering the verbal support for experiential avoidance. *The Behavior Analyst, 17*, 289-303.

Hayes, S. C., Wilson, K. G., Gifford, E. V., Bissett, R., Piasecki, M., Batten, S. V., et al. (2004). A randomized controlled trial of twelve-step facilitation and acceptance and commitment therapy with polysubstance abusing methadone maintained opiate addicts. *Behavior Therapy, 35*, 667-688.

Hayes, S. C., Wilson, K. G., Gifford, E. V., Follette, V. M., & Strosahl, K. (1996). Emotional avoidance and behavioral disorders: A functional dimensional approach to diagnosis and treatment. *Journal of Consulting and Clinical Psychology, 64*, 1152-1168.

Heffner, M., & Eifert, G. H. (2004). *The anorexia workbook: How to accept yourself, heal suffering, and reclaim your life*. Oakland, CA: New Harbinger.

Heijden, G., van der Beurskens, A., Dirx, M., Bouter, L., & Lindeman, E. (1995). Efficacy of lumbar traction: a randomized clinical trial. *Physiotherapy, 81*, 29-35.

Herzog, W., Conway, P., & Willcox, B. (1991). Effects of different treatment modalities on gait symmetry and clinical measures for sacroiliac joint patients. *Journal of Manipulative Physiological Therapeutics, 14*, 104-109.

Hickey, R. (1982). Chronic low back pain: a comparison of diflunisal with paracetamol. *New Zealand Medical Journal, 5*, 312-314.

Hides, J., Richardson, C., & Jull, G. (1995). Magnetic resonance imaging and ultrasonography of the lumbar multifidus muscle: Comparison of two different modalities. *Spine, 20*, 54-58.

Hides, J., Richardson, C., & Jull, G. (1996). Multifidus muscle recovery is not automatic after resolution of acute, first-episode low back pain. *Spine, 21*(23), 2763-2769.

Hides, J., Stokes, M., & Saide, M. (1994). Evidence of lumbar multifidus muscle wasting ipsilateral to symptoms in patients with acute/subacute low back pain. *Spine, 19*, 165-172.

Horvath, A. O., & Luborsky, L. (1993). The role of the therapeutic alliance in psychotherapy. *Journal of Consulting and Clinical Psychology, 61*, 561-573.

Houlihan, D., Rodriguez, H. D., & Kloeckl, J. (1990). Validation of a reinforcer survey for use with geriatric patients. *Behavioral Residential Treatment, 5*, 129-136.

Hurri, H. (1989a). The Swedish back school in chronic low-back pain. Part I. *Scandinavian Journal of Rehabilitation Medicine, 21*, 33-40.

Hurri, H. (1989b). The Swedish back school in chronic low-back pain. Part II. *Scandinavian Journal of Rehabilitation Medicine, 21*, 41-44.

Jensen, I., Nygren, Å., & Lundin, A. (1994). Cognitive-behavioral treatment for workers with chronic spinal pain: A matched and controlled cohort study in Sweden. *Occupational and Environmental Medicine, 51*, 145-151.

Jensen, I., & Bodin, L. (1998). Multimodal cognitive-behavioral treatment for workers with chronic spinal pain: A matched cohort study with an 18-month follow-up. *Pain, 76*, 35-44.

Johannisson, K. (1997). *Kroppens tunna skal* (The thin skin of the body). Stockholm: Norstedts.

Johansson, E. (1998) Beyond Frustration: Understanding women with undefined musculoskeletal pain who consult primary care. Doctoral dissertation, Umeå University (550) ISSN 03546-6612.

Johansson, E., Hamberg, K., Lindgren, G., & Westman, G. (1999). The meanings of pain: A qualitative exploration of symptom description in a group of female patients with long term musculoskeletal disorders. *Social Science Medicine, 48*, 1791-1802.

Johansson, E., Hamberg, K., Lindgren, G., & Westman, G. (1999). The meanings of pain: A qualitative exploration of symptom descriptions in a group of female patients with long-term musculoskeletal disorders. *Social Science Medicine, 48*, 1791-1802.

Kabat-Zinn, J. (1990). *Full catastrophe living: Using the wisdom of your body and mind to face stress, pain, and illness.* New York: Delacorte Press.

Karekla, M., Forsyth, J. P., & Kelly, M. M. (2004). Emotional avoidance and panicogenic responding to a biological challenge procedure. *Behavior Therapy, 35*, 725-746.

Keijsers, J., Steenbakkers, W., Meertens, R., Bouter, L., & Kok, G. (1990). The efficacy of the back school: A randomized trial. *Arthritis Care and Research, 3*, 204-209.

Keller, S., Ehrhardt-Schmelzer, S., Herda, C., Schmid, S., & Basler, H. (1997). Multidisciplinary rehabilitation for chronic back pain in an outpatient setting: A controlled randomized trial. *European Journal of Pain, 1*, 279-292.

Kendall, P., & Jenkins, J. (1968). Exercises for backache: a double-blind controlled trial. *Physiotherapy, 54*, 154-157.

Kerns, R., Turk, D., Holzman, A., & Rudy, T. (1986). Comparison of cognitive behavioral and behavioral approaches to the outpatient treatment of chronic pain. *Clinical Journal of Pain, 1*, 195-203.

King, A., & Cavanaugh, J. (1996). Neurophysiologic basis of low back pain. In S. Wiesel, J. Weinstein, H. Herkowitz, J. Dvorak, & G. Bell (Eds.), *The lumbar spine* (2nd ed., pp. 74-85). Philadelphia: Saunders.

Klaber-Moffett, J., Chase, S., Portek. I., & Ennis, J. (1986). A controlled prospective study to evaluate the effectiveness of a back school in the relief of chronic low-back pain. *Spine, 11,* 120-122.

Klienman, A. (1988). *The illness narratives; suffering, healing, and the human condition.* New York: Basic Books.

Koes, B. W., Bouter, L. M., & van Mameren, H. (1993). A randomized clinical trial of manual therapy and physiotherapy for persistent back and neck complaints: Subgroups analysis and relationship between outcome measures. *Journal of Manipulative Physiological Therapeutics, 16,* 211-219.

Koes, B. W., Bouter, L. M., van Mameren, H., Essers, A. H., Verstegen, G., Hofhizen, D. M., et al. (1992a). A blinded randomized clinical trial of manual therapy and physiotherapy for chronic back and neck complaints: Physical outcome measures. *Journal of Manipulative Physiological Therapeutics, 15,* 16-23.

Koes, B. W., Bouter, L. M., van Mameren, H., Essers, A. H., Verstegen, G. H., Hofuizen, D. M., et al. (1992b). The effectiveness of manual therapy, physiotherapy and treatment by the general practitioner for non-specific back and neck complaints: A randomized clinical trial. *Spine, 17,* 28-35.

Koes, B. W., Bouter, L. M., van Mameren, H., Essers, A. H., Verstegen, G. M., Hofhuizen, D. M., et al. (1992c). Randomized clinical trial of manipulative therapy and physiotherapy for persistent back and neck complaints: Results of one year follow-up. *British Medical Journal, 304,* 601-605.

Kral, B., Becker, L., Blumenthal, R., Aversano, T., Fleisher, L., Yook, R., et al. (1997). Exaggerated reactivity to mental stress is associated with exercise-induced myocardial ischemia in an asymptomatic high-risk population. *Circulation, 96,* 4246-4253.

Krause, J. (1992). Spinal cord injury and its rehabilitation. *Current Opinions Neurology and Neurosurgery, 5,* 669-672.

Lankhorst, G., van der Stadt, R., Vogelaar, T., van der Korst, J., & Prevo, A. (1983). The effect of the Swedish back school in chronic idiopathic low-back pain. *Scandinavian Journal of Rehabilitation Medicine, 15,* 141-145.

Lee, C., & Powers, J. (2002). Number of social roles, health and well-being: Three generations of Australian women. *International Journal of Behavioral Medicine, 9,* 195-215.

Lehmann, T., Russell, D., & Spratt, K. (1983). The impact of patients with nonorganic physical findings on a controlled trial of TENS and electroacupunture. *Spine, 8,* 625-634.

Lehmann, T. R., Russell, D. W., Spratt, K. F., Colby, H., King Liu, Y., Fairchild, M., et al. (1986). Efficacy of electroacuupuncture and TENS in the rehabilitation of chronic low back pain patients. *Pain, 26*(3), 277-290.

Leijon, M., Hensing, G., & Alexanderson, K. (1998). Gender trends in sick-listing with musculoskeletal symptoms in a Swedish county during a period of rapid increase in sickness absence. *Scandinavian Journal of Social Medicine, 26,* 204-213.

Leijon, M., Hensing, G., & Alexanderson, K., (1998). Gender trends in sick listing with musculoskeletal symptoms in a Swedish county during a period of rapid increase in sickness absence. *Scandinavian Journal of Social Medicine, 26*, 204-213

Leitenberg, H., Greenwald, E., & Cado, S. (1992). A retrospective study of longterm methods of coping with having been sexually abused during childhood. *Child Abuse and Neglect, 16*, 399-407.

Levitt, J. T., Brown, T. A., Orsillo, S. M., & Barlow, D. H. (2004). The effects of acceptance versus suppression of emotion on subjective and psychophysiological response to carbon dioxide challenge in patients with panic disorder. *Behavior Therapy, 35*, 747-766.

Lindström, I., Öhlund, C., Eek, C., Wallin, L., Peterson, L-E., Fordyce, W., et al. (1992). The effect of graded activity on patients with subacute low back pain: A randomized prospective clinical study with an operant conditioning behavior approach. *Physical Therapy, 72*, 279-293.

Lindström, I., Öhlund, C., Eek, C., Wallin, L., Peterson, L-E., & Nachemsom, A. (1992). Mobility, strength, and fitness after a graded activity program for patients with subacute low back pain. *Spine, 17*, 641-652.

Lindström, I., & Zachrisson, M. (1970). Physical therapy on low back pain and sciatica: an attempt at evaluation. *Scandinavian Journal of Rehabilitation Medicine, 2*, 37-42.

Linton, S. (2000). Psykologiska faktorers betydelse *[Psychological factors in pain]*. I SBU-rapport, *Ont i ryggen, ont i nacken [Pain in back, pain in neck]*, vol. I (pp. 117-155). Stockholm: SBU.

Linton, S. (2002). Early identification and intervention in the prevention of musculoskeletal pain. *American Journal of Industrial Medicine, 41*, 433-442.

Linton, S., Bradley, L., Jensen, I., & Sundell, L. (1989). The secondary prevention of low-back pain. A controlled study with follow-up. *Pain, 36*, 197-207.

Linton, S., & Buer, N. (1995). Working despite pain: Factors associated with work attendance versus dysfunction. *International Journal of Behavioral Medicine, 2*, 252-262.

Linton, S., & Götestam, K. G. (1984). A controlled study of the effects of applied relaxation and applied relaxation plus operant procedures on the regulation of chronic pain. *British Journal of Clinical Psychology, 23*, 291-299.

Linton, S., & Hallden, K. (1998). Interpretation of abnormal illness behavior in low back pain. *Pain, 39*, 41-53.

Linton, S., Melin, L., & Sternlöf, K. (1985). The effects of applied relaxation and operant activity training on chronic pain. *Behavioral Psychotherapy, 13*, 87-100.

Loisel, P., Abenhaim, L., Durand, P., Esdaile, J., Suissa, S., Gosselin, L. et al. (1997). A population-based randomized clinical trial on back pain management. *Spine, 22*(24), 2911-2918.

Luciano, C., & Hayes, S. C. (2001). Trastorno de Evitación Experiential [Experiential Avoidance Disorder]. *International Journal of Clinical and Health Psychology, 1*(1), 109-157.

Luciano, C., Rodriguez, M., & Guitierrez, O. (2004). Synthesizing verbal contexts in experiential avoidance disorder. *Journal of Psychology and Psychological Therapy*, 4(2), 377-394.

Lundberg, U. (1996). Influence of paid and unpaid work on psychophysiological stress response of men and women. *Journal of Occupational Health Psychology*, 1, 117-130.

Lundberg, U., Mårderg, B., & Frankenhauser, M. (1994). The total workload of male and female white-collar workers as related to age, occupation level, and number of children. *Scandinavian Journal of Psychology*, 35, 315-327.

MacDonald, A., MacRae, K., Master, B., & Rubin, A. (1983). Superficial acupuncture in the relief of low back pain. *Annuals of Royal College of Surgery in England*, 65, 44-46.

Manniche, C., Asmussen, K., Lauritsen, B., Vinterberg, H., Karbo, H., Abildstrup, S., et al. (1993). Intensive dynamic back exercises with or without hyperextension in chronic back pain after surgery for lumbar disc protrusion: a clinical trial. *Spine*, 18, 560-567.

Manniche, C., Hesselsoe, G., Bentzen, L., Christensen, I., & Lundberg, E. (1988). Clinical trial of intensive muscle training for chronic low back pain. *Lancet*, 2, 1473-1476.

Manniche, C., Lundberg, E., Christensen, I., Bentzen, L., & Hesselsoe, G. (1991). Intensive dynamic back exercises for chronic low back pain: A clinical trial. *Pain*, 47, 53-63.

Marchand, S, Charest, J., Li, J., Chenard, J., Lavignolle, B., & Laurencelle, L. (1993). In TENS purely a placebo effect? A controlled study on chronic low back pain. *Pain*, 54, 99-106.

Martin, P., Rose, M., Nichols, P., Russell, P., & Hughes, J. (1980). Physiotherapy exercises for low back pain: Process and clinical outcome. *International Journal of Rehabilitation Medicine*, 8, 34-38.

Masuda, A., Hayes, S. C., Sackett, C. F., & Twohig, M. P. (2004). Cognitive defusion and self-relevant negative thoughts: Examining the impact of a ninety year old technique. *Behaviour Research and Therapy*, 42, 477-485.

Matsumo, S., Kaneda, K., & Nohara, Y. (1991). Clinical evaluation of Ketoprofen, (orudis) in lumbago: A double blind comparison with Dicloefenac Sodium. *British Journal of Clinical Practice*, 35, 266.

Mayou, R., & Sharpe, M. (1997). Treating medically unexplained physical symptoms. Effective interventions are available. *British Medical Journal*, 315, 561-562.

McCracken, L. M. (1998). Learning to live with the pain: Acceptance of pain predicts adjustment in persons with chronic pain. *Pain*, 74, 21-27.

McCracken, L. M., & Eccleston, C. (2003). Coping or acceptance: What to do about chronic pain. *Pain*, 105, 197-204.

McCracken, L. M., Vowles, K. E., & Eccleston, C. (2004). Acceptance of chronic pain: Component analysis and a revised assessment method. *Pain*, 107, 159-166.

McCracken, L. M., Vowles, K. E., & Eccleston, C. (in press). Acceptance-based treatment for persons with complex, long-standing chronic pain: A preliminary analysis of treatment outcome in comparison to a waiting phase. *Behaviour Research and Therapy.*

Melamed, S., Grosswasser, Z., & Stern, M. (1992). Acceptance of disability, work, involvement and subjective rehabilitation status of traumatic brain-injured (TBI) patients. *Brain Injury, 6,* 233-243.

Mendelson, G., Kidson, M., Loh, S., Scott, D., Selwood, T., & Kranz, H. (1978). Acupuncture analgesia for chronic low back pain. *Clinical Experimental Neurology, 15,* 182-185.

Mendelson, G., Selwood, T., Kranz, H., Loh, S., Kidson, M., & Scott, D. (1983). Acupuncture treatment of chronic low back pain. *American Journal of Medicine, 74,* 49-55.

Merskey, H., & Bogduk, N. (Eds.). (1994). *Classification of chronic pain: Descriptions of chronic pain syndromes and definitions of pain terms* (2nd ed.). Seattle: IASP.

Million, R., Nilsen, K., Jayson, M., & Baker, R. (1981). Evaluation of low-back pain and assessment of lumbar corsets with and without back support. *Annual of Rheumatic Disorders, 40,* 449-454.

Mitchell, R., & Carmen, G. (1994). The functional restoration approach to the treatment of chronic pain in patients with soft tissue and back injuries. *Spine, 19,* 635-642.

Mixter, W., & Barr, J. (1934). Rupture of the intervertebral disc with involvement of the spinal canal. *New England Medical Journal, 211,* 210-215.

Moen, P., Erickson, M., & Dempster-McClain, D. (2000). Social role identities among older adults in a continuing care retirement community. *Research on aging, 22,* 559-579.

Molsberger, A., Winkler, J., Schneider, S., & Mau, J. (1998). Acupuncture and conventional orthopedic pain treatment in the management of chronic low back pain: a prospective randomized and controlled clinical trial. *Proceedings of the ISSLS, 6,* 87.

Moore, J., & Chaney, E. (1985). Outpatient group treatment of chronic pain: Effects of spouse involvement. *Journal of Consulting and Clinical Psychology, 53,* 326-334.

Moore, J., Von Korff, M., Cherkin, D., Saunders, K., & Lorig, K. (2000). A randomized trial of a cognitive-behavioral program for enhancing back pain self care in a primary setting. *Pain, 88,* 145-153.

Moore, S., & Shurman, J. (1997). Combined neuromuscular electrical stimulation and transcutaneous electrical nerve stimulation for treatment of chronic back pain: a double blind, repeated measures comparison. *Archives of Physical Medical Rehabilitation, 78,* 55-60.

Morley, S., Eccleston, C., & Williams, A. (1999). Systematic review and meta-analysis of randomized controlled trials of cognitive behavior therapy for chronic pain in adults excluding headache. *Pain, 80,* 1-13.

Moser, A. E., & Annis, H. M. (1996). The role of coping in relapse crisis outcome: A prospective study of treated alcoholics. *Addiction, 91*(8), 1101-1114.

Nachemson, A., & Jonsson, E. (2000). Inledning [Introduction]. I SBU-rapport, *Ont i ryggen, ont i nacken [Pain in back, pain in neck]*, vol. I (pp. 33-43) Stockholm: SBU.

Nachemson, G., & Waddell, H. (2000). Förekomst av smärta I nacken och ländryggen *[Prevalence of pain in the neck and low back]*. I SBU-rapport, *Ont i ryggen, ont i nacken [Pain in back, pain in neck]*, vol. I (pp. 311-389). Stockholm: SBU.

National Alliance for Care giving and the American Association of Retired Persons. (1997). *Family care-giving in the US: Findings from a national survey*. Bethesda, MD: NAC/AARP.

Newton-John, T., Spence, S., & Schotte, D. (1995). Cognitive behavior therapy versus EMG biofeedback in the treatment of chronic low back pain. *Behavior Research Therapy, 33*, 691-697.

Nicholas, M., Wilson, P., & Goyen, J. (1991). Operant-behavioral and cognitive behvavioral treatment for chronic low back pain. *Behavior Research and Therapy, 29*, 225-238.

Nicholas, M., Wilson, P., & Goyen, J. (1992). Comparison of a cognitive-behavioral group treatment and an alternative non-psychological treatment for chronic low back pain. *Pain, 48*, 339-347.

Nouwen, A. (1983). EMG biofeedback used to reduce standing levels of paraspinal muscle tension in chronic low back pain. *Pain, 17*, 353-360.

Ogden, J. (1997). The rhetoric and reality of psychosocial theories of health. *Journal of Health Psychology, 2*, 21-29.

Olson, A., Hansen, H., & Eriksson, H. (1993). I Rapport till expertgruppen för studier I offentlig ekonomi, [*Social Security in Sweden and other European Countries–Three essays*]. Ds, 1993:51. Stockholm: Financial Department.

Ongley, M., Klein, R., Dorman, T., Eek, B., & Hubert, L. (1987). A new approach to the treatment of chronic low back pain. *Lancet, 8551*, 143-146.

Orth-Gomer, K. (1998). Psychosocial risk factor profile in women with coronary heart disease. In K. Orth-Gomer, & M. Chesney (Eds.), *Women, stress and heart disease* (pp. 25-40). Mahwah, NJ: Lawrence Erlbaum.

Paez, M., Luciano, C., Gutierrez, O., & Rodriguez, M. (2005). *Experimental pain task in the context of values*. Paper presented in a symposium for the Association of Behavior Analysis, Chicago, 2005.

Papageorgiou, A., Croft, P., Ferry, S., Jayson, M., & Sliman, A. (1995). Estimating the prevalence of low back pain in the general population: Evidence from the South Manchester back pain survey. *Spine, 20*, 1889-1894.

Park, J., & Liao, T. (2000). The effects of multiple roles of South Korean married women professors: Role changes and the factors that influence potential role gratification and strain. *Sex Roles, 43*, 571-591.

Parson, T. (1951). *The social system*. New York: Free Press.

Peters, J., & Large, R. (1990). A randomized control trial evaluating in and out-patient management programs. *Pain, 41*, 283-289.

Polusny, M. A., & Follette, V. M. (1995). Long-term correlates of child sexual abuse: Theory and review of the empirical literature. *Applied and Preventive Psychology, 4,* 143-166.

Postacchini, F., Facchini, M., & Palieri, P. (1988). Efficacy of various forms of conservative treatment in low back pain: A comparative study. *Neurological Orthopedic, 6,* 28-35.

Puder, R. (1988). Age analysis of cognitive behavioral group therapy for chronic pain outpatients. *Psychology and Aging, 3,* 204-207.

Purdon, C. (1999). Thought suppression and psychopathology. *Behaviour Research and Therapy, 37,* 1029-1054.

Raspe, H. (1993). Back pain. In A. Silman & M. C. Hoch (Eds.), *Epidemiology of the rheumatic diseases* (pp. 330-374). Oxford: Oxford University Press.

Reifman, A., Biernat, B., & Lang, E. (1991). Stress, social support and health in married professional women with small children. *Psychology of Women Quarterly, 15,* 431-445.

Ridley, M., Kingsley, G., Gibson, T., & Grahame, R. (1988). Outpatient lumbar epidural corticosteroid injection in the management of sciatica. *British Journal of Rheumatology, 27,* 295-299.

Riegal, B. (1993). Contributors to cardiac invalidism after acute myocardial infarction. *Coronary Artery Diseases, 4,* 215-220.

Risch, S., Norvell, N., Pollock, M., Risch, E., Langer, H., Fulton, M., et al. (1993). Lumbar strengthening in chronic low back pain patients, physiologic and psychological benefits. *Spine, 18*(2), 232-238.

Robinson, P., & Hayes, S. C. (1997). Acceptance and commitment: A model for integration. In N. A. Cummings, J. L. Cummings, & J. A. Johnsson (Eds.), *Behavioral health in primary care: A guide for clinical integration* (pp.177-203). Madison, CT: Psychosocial Press.

Robinson, P., & Hayes, S. C. (1997). Acceptance and Commitment: A model for integration. In N. Cummings, J. Cummings, & J. Johnsson (Eds.), *Behavioral health in primary care: A guide to clinical integration* (pp. 177-203). Madison, CT: Psychosocial Press.

Rocco, A., Frank, E., Kaul, A., Lipson, S., & Gallo, J. (1989). Epidural morphine and epidural steroids combined with morphine in the treatment of post laminectomy syndrome. *Pain, 36,* 297-303.

Rydh, J. (2002). Handlingsplan for ökad hälsa I arbetslivet (Action plan for improved health in the working life). *The Swedish Council on Heath, Technology and Assessment in Health Care,* Vol. 5. Stockholm: SBU.

Sachs, B., Ahmad, S., la Croix, M., Olimpio, D., Heath, R., David, J. A., et al. (1994). Objective assessment for exercise treatment on the B-200 isostation as part of work tolerance rehabilitation: A random prospective blind evaluation with comparison control population. *Spine, 19*(1), 49-52.

Saunders, K., Von Korff, M., & Grothaus, L. (2000). Predictors of participation in primary care group-format back pain self-care intervention. *Clinical Journal of Pain, 16,* 236-243.

SCB (1996). *Statistics Sweden: National household surveys.* Stockholm: SCB

Serrao, J., Marks, R., Morely, S., & Goodchild, C. (1999). Intrathe-cal midazolam for the treatment of chronic mechanical low back pain: A controlled comparison with epidural steroid in a pilot study. *Pain, 48,* 5-12.

Siegmeth, W., & Sieberer, W. (1978). A comparison of the short-term effects of ibuprofen and diclofenas in spondylois. *Journal of internal Medical Research, 6,* 369-374.

Skekelle, P. (1997). The epidemiology of low back pain. In L. Giles & K. Singer (Eds.), *Clinical anatomy and management of low back pain* (pp. 18-31). London: Butterworth Heinemann.

Skinner, B. F. (1974). *About behaviorism.* New York: Vintage Books.

Skovron, M., Szpalski, M., Nordin, M., Melot, C., & Cukier, D. (1994). Sociocultural factors and back pain: A population-based study in Belgian adults. *Spine, 19,* 129-137.

Spence, S. (1989). Cognitive behavior therapy in the management of chronic, occupational pain of the upper limbs. *Behavior Research and Therapy, 27,* 435-446.

Spence, S., Sharp, L., Newton-John, T., & Champion, D. (1995). Effects of EMG biofeedback compared to applied relaxation training with chronic upper extremity cumulative trauma disorders. *Pain, 63,* 199-206.

Stevens, M., & Franks, M. (1999). Parent care in the context of woman's multiple roles. *Current directions in Psychological Science, 8,* 149-152.

Strong, J. (1998). Incorporating cognitive-behavior therapy with occupational therapy: A comparative study with patients with low back pain. *Journal of Occupational Rehabilitation, 8,* 61-71.

Strosahl, K. D., Hayes, S. C., Wilson, K. G., & Gifford, E. V. (2004). An ACT primer: Core therapy processes, intervention strategies, and therapist competencies. In S. C. Hayes & K. D. Strosahl (Eds.), *A practical guide to Acceptance and Commitment Therapy* (pp. 31-58). New York: Kluwer/Plenum.

Stuckey, S., Jacobs, A., & Goldfarb, J. (1986). EMG biofeedback training, relaxation training, and placebo for the relief of chronic low back pain. *Perceptive Motor Skills, 63,* 1023-1036.

Svensson, H., & Brorson, J. (1997). Sweden, Sickness and work injury insurance, a summary of developments. *International Social Security Review, 50,* 75-86.

Takahashi, M., Muto, T., Tada, M., & Sugiyama, M. (2002). Acceptance rationale and increasing pain tolerance: Acceptance-based and FEAR-based practice. *Japanese Journal of Behavior Therapy, 28,* 35-46.

Taylor, H., & Curran, N. (1985). *The Nuprin Pain Report.* New York: Louis Harris and Associates.

Triano, J., McGregor, M., Hondras, M., & Brennan, P. (1995). Manipulative therapy versus education programs in chronic low-back pain. *Spine, 20,* 948-955.

Turk, D., & Rudy, T. E. (1989). A cognitive-behavioral perspective on chronic pain: Beyond the scalpel and syringe. In C. D. Tollison (Ed.), *Handbook of chronic pain management* (pp. 222-236). Baltimore: Williams & Wilkins.

Turner, J., & Jensen, M. (1993). Efficacy of cognitive therapy for chronic low back pain. *Pain, 52,* 169-177.

Turner, J. (1996). Educational and behavioral interventions for back pain in primary care. *Spine, 21,* 2851-2859.

Turner, J., Clancy, S., McQuade, K., & Cardenas, D. (1984). Effectiveness of behavioral therapy for chronic low back pain, a component analysis. *Journal of Consulting Clinical Psychology, 52,* 169-177.

Turner, J., Clancy, S., McQuade, K., & *Cardenas*, D. (1990). Effectiveness of behavior therapy for chronic low back pain: A component analysis. *Journal of Consulting and Clinical Psychology, 58,* 573-579.

Van Tulder, M., Goossens, M., & Nachemson, A. (2000). Kroniska ländryggsbesvär-konservativ behandling*[Chronic low back pain-conservative treatment]* . I SBU-rapport, *Ont i ryggen, ont i nacken [Pain in back, pain in neck],* vol. II (pp. 17-113). Stockholm: SBU.

Van Tulder, M., Koes, B., & Bouter, L. (1997). Conservative treatment of acute and chronic non-specific low back pain. *Spine, 22,* 2128-2156.

Vendrig, A. (1999). Prognostic factors and treatment-related changes associated with return to work in the multimodal treatment of chronic back pain. *Journal of Behavior Medicine, 22,* 217-232.

Videman, T., & Osterman, K. (1984). Double blind parallel study of Piroxicam versus Idomethacin in the treatment of low back pain. *Annals of Clinical Research, 16,* 156-160.

Von Korff, M., Moore, J., Lorig, K., Cherkin, D., Saunders, K., & Gonzalez, V. (1998). A randomized trial of a lay-led self-management group intervention for back pain patients in primary care. *Spine, 23,* 2608-2615.

Waagen, G., Haldeman, S., Cook, G., Lopez, D., & DeBoer, K. (1986). Short-term trial of chiropractic adjustments for the relief of chronic low back pain. *Manual Medicine, 2,* 63-67.

Waddell, G. (1991). Low back disability: A syndrome of western civilization. *Neurosurgery Clinics of North America, 2,* 719-738.

Waddell, G., & Norlund, A. (2000). System för socialförsäkring en internationell jämförelse (System for health insurance: An international comparison). I SBU-rapport, *Ont i ryggen, ont i nacken [Pain in back, pain in neck],* (pp. 311-389). Stockholm: SBU.

Waddell, G., Pilowsky, I., & Bond, M., (1989). Clinical assessment and interpretation of abnormal illness behavior in low back pain. *Pain, 39,* 41-53.

Waddell, G., & Waddell, H. (2000). Sociala faktorers inflytande (The influence of social factors). I SBU-rapport, *Ont i ryggen, ont i nacken [Pain in back, pain in neck],* vol. I (pp. 51-116). Stockholm: SBU.

Walsh, K., Cruddas, M., & Coggon, D. (1992). Low back pain in eight areas of Britain. *Journal of Epidemiology and Community Heath, 46,* 227-230.

Wegner, D. M. (1994). *White bears and other unwanted thoughts: Suppression, obsession, and the psychology of mental control.* New York: Guilford.

Wegner, D. M., Schneider, D. J., Carter, S. R., & White, T. L. (1987). Paradoxical effects of thought suppression. *Journal of Personality and Social Psychology, 53,* 5-13.

Wegner, D. M., Schneider, D. J., Knutson, B., & McMahon, S. R. (1991). Polluting the stream of consciousness: The effect of thought suppression on the mind's environment. *Cognitive Therapy and Research, 15,* 141-152.

White, A. (1966). Low back pain in men receiving workmen's compensation. *Canadian Medical Association Journal, 95,* 50-56.

Wiesel, S., Tsourmas, N., Feffer, H., Citrin, C., & Patronas, N. (1984). A study of computer-assisted tomography. I. The incidence of positive CAT scans in an asymptomatic group of patients. *Spine, 9,* 549-551.

Williams, A., Richardson, P., & Nicholas, M., (1996). Inpatient versus outpatient pain management: Results of a randomized controlled trial. *Pain, 66,* 13-22.

Wilson, K. G., & Blackledge, J .T. (2000). A behavior analytic analysis of language: Making sense of clinical phenomenon. In M. G. Dougher (Ed.), *Clinical behavior analysis* (pp. 47-74). Reno, NV: Context Press.

Wilson, K. G., & Groom, J. (2002). *The Valued Living Questionnaire.* Available from the first author at Department of Psychology, University of Mississippi, University, MS.

Wilson, K. G., Hayes, S. C., Gregg, J., & Zettle, R. D. (2001). Psychopathology and psychotherapy. In S. C. Hayes, D. Barnes, & B. Roche (Eds.), *Relational Frame Theory: A Post Skinnerian account of human language and cognition* (pp. 211-237). New York: Plenum Press.

Wilson, K. G., & Luciano, C. (2002). Terapia de Aceptación y Compromiso [ACT]. Un tratamiento conductual orientado a los valores. Madrid: Pirámide.

Wilson, K. G., & Murrell, A. R. (2004). Values work in Acceptance and Commitment Therapy: Setting a course for behavioral treatment. In S. C. Hayes, V. M. Follette, & M. Linehan (Eds.), *Mindfulness and acceptance: Expanding the cognitive behavioral tradition* (pp. 120-151). New York: Guilford.

Wolf, F., Ross, K., Anderson, J., Russell, I. J., & Herbert, L. (1995). The prevalence and characteristics of fibromyalgia in the general population. *Arthritis Rheumatology, 38,* 19-28.